Internet of Things and Machine Learning

Series Editor: Dr. Vishal Jain, Sharda University, Greater Noida, India
Email: drvishaljain83@gmail.com

Technology is moving at an exponential pace in this modern era of computational intelligence. To complement this, Internet of Things and Machine Learning have emerged most promising tool for researchers and innovators to challenge themselves and think beyond the walls about new possibilities. The dependency of human processes on machine learning driven systems is encompassing all spheres of current state of the art systems. There is a huge potential in this domain to make the best use of machines in order to ensure the optimal prediction, execution and decision making. For this series, we invite researchers, academicians and professionals to contribute chapters expressing their ideas and research in the application of intelligent techniques to the field of engineering. Both theoretical contributions and practical applications in the area of intelligent techniques are welcome. This series shall help clarify understanding of certain key mechanisms and technologies helpful in realizing such systems.

nova
science publishers
www.novapublishers.com

Internet of Things and Machine Learning

Artificial Intelligence and Digital Diversity Inclusiveness in Corporate Restructuring
Richa Goel, PhD, S. K. Baral, PhD, Ramamurthy Venkatesh, PhD
2022. ISBN: 978-1-68507-786-0 (Hardcover)
2022. ISBN: 979-8-88697-074-6 (eBook)

Intelligent Information Retrieval for Healthcare Systems
Ankur Choudhary, PhD, Arun Prakash Agrawal, PhD, Parma Nand, PhD, Vishal Jain, PhD
2021. ISBN: 978-1-68507-301-5 (Hardcover)
2021. ISBN: 978-1-68507-365-7 (eBook)

Internet of Things and Machine Learning in Agriculture
Jyotir Moy Chatterjee (Editor)
Vishal Jain, PhD
2021. ISBN: 978-1-68507-192-9 (Hardcover)
2021. ISBN: 978-1-68507-216-2 (eBook)

Machine Learning Algorithms Using Python Programming
Gopal Sakarkar, PhD (Author)
2021. ISBN: 978-1-53619-512-5 (Softcover)
2021. ISBN: 978-1-53619-615-3 (eBook)

More information about this series can be found at
https://novapublishers.com/product-category/series/internet-of-things-and-machine-learning/

Internet of Things and Machine Learning

Series Editor: Dr. Vishal Jain, Sharda University, Greater Noida, India
Email: drvishaljain83@gmail.com

Technology is moving at an exponential pace in this modern era of computational intelligence. To complement this, Internet of Things and Machine Learning have emerged most promising tool for researchers and innovators to challenge themselves and think beyond the walls about new possibilities. The dependency of human processes on machine learning driven systems is encompassing all spheres of current state of the art systems. There is a huge potential in this domain to make the best use of machines in order to ensure the optimal prediction, execution and decision making. For this series, we invite researchers, academicians and professionals to contribute chapters expressing their ideas and research in the application of intelligent techniques to the field of engineering. Both theoretical contributions and practical applications in the area of intelligent techniques are welcome. This series shall help clarify understanding of certain key mechanisms and technologies helpful in realizing such systems.

nova
science publishers

www.novapublishers.com

Internet of Things and Machine Learning

Artificial Intelligence and Digital Diversity Inclusiveness in Corporate Restructuring
Richa Goel, PhD, S. K. Baral, PhD, Ramamurthy Venkatesh, PhD
2022. ISBN: 978-1-68507-786-0 (Hardcover)
2022. ISBN: 979-8-88697-074-6 (eBook)

Intelligent Information Retrieval for Healthcare Systems
Ankur Choudhary, PhD, Arun Prakash Agrawal, PhD, Parma Nand, PhD, Vishal Jain, PhD
2021. ISBN: 978-1-68507-301-5 (Hardcover)
2021. ISBN: 978-1-68507-365-7 (eBook)

Internet of Things and Machine Learning in Agriculture
Jyotir Moy Chatterjee (Editor)
Vishal Jain, PhD
2021. ISBN: 978-1-68507-192-9 (Hardcover)
2021. ISBN: 978-1-68507-216-2 (eBook)

Machine Learning Algorithms Using Python Programming
Gopal Sakarkar, PhD (Author)
2021. ISBN: 978-1-53619-512-5 (Softcover)
2021. ISBN: 978-1-53619-615-3 (eBook)

More information about this series can be found at
https://novapublishers.com/product-category/series/internet-of-things-and-machine-learning/

Tawseef Ayoub Shaikh, Tabasum Rasool and Mohammed Wasid
Editors

AI-Enabled IoT for Smart Health Care Systems

nova
science publishers
www.novapublishers.com

DOI: https://doi.org/10.52305/RGPB8318

Library of Congress Cataloging-in-Publication Data

ISBN: 978-1-68507-977-2

Published by Nova Science Publishers, Inc. † New York

Dedication

To my wonderful parents, Haji Mohd Ayoub Shaikh and Kulsoomah Banoo

—Tawseef Ayoub Shaikh

To my beloved parents for their patience, love, and support throughout my career

—Tabasum Rasool

To my beloved parents

—Mohammed Wasid

Contents

Preface

Rapid developments in automated data collecting methods in clinical sciences have resulted in a tsunami of patient-specific data being stored in scattered, heterogeneous, huge databases and datamarts. The lack of existing computing tools to enable connectivity and interoperability between these fragmented sources and scattered locations (access issues) and to perform machine learning on heterogeneous and highly dimensional data sources (complexity issues) is a crippling impediment, not only to health care but also to computational research. Furthermore, the rapid deployment of high-speed networks, combined with advances in knowledge discovery aided by mobile technologies, has heightened the urgent need for a unified, coherent computing infrastructure to support, enhance, and empower multi-disciplinary and multi-institutional health care informatics research. Health care data is complex, context-dependent, intrinsically heterogeneous, and high-dimensional, posing a slew of computing research problems that make extracting useful knowledge from raw data a difficult computational endeavour. These data resources cover a wide range of data formats, from simple text notes to complicated image types like positron emission tomography images.

More complicated data types, such as hyperspectral imaging, are becoming more readily available as clinical data collection technology advances and storage prices fall. These diversified and abundant data sources serve as an excellent research testbed for the development of novel machine learning algorithms, which are at the heart of the current data-rich but information-poor paradigm, which affects a wide range of fields beyond health care. It is evident that an integrated, panoramic view of data will provide an opportunity for previously impossible clinical insights and discoveries. Machine learning and analytics have the potential to restore "care" to health care by augmenting human performance. One of the most important topics is health care. Finding relevant information is a crucial effort. The patient is now at the centre of the health care ecosystem, thanks to machine learning and health analytics. Patients, who are looking for ways to improve their wellbeing and health, have access to a variety of technological elements, with machine learning and analytics at the forefront. The health-related data are also handled at a lightning speed. The onus is to find nuggets of information from this vast ocean of data, which is unlikely to be achieved without these cutting-edge technologies.

Furthermore, machine learning and analytics are being integrated into all the sectors generating huge numbers of data points every day. This edited book covers all aspects of the machine learning techniques and applications, with a complete 360-degree view. This book seeks to close the gap between engineering and medicine, combining health sciences with the design and problem-solving skills of engineering to advance health care treatments, including diagnosis, monitoring, and therapy. Health plays such a vital role in our lives that health care management becomes an essential part of society. Traditionally, health care was considered to be the domain of only medical practitioners. But, as the 'digital age' has approached, the medical field has become digitized too. Machine learning and analytics have given wings to the health care industry. Health care solutions, when powered by machine learning and analytics, increase as well as deepen. Several case studies, combining machine learning with health care, are also incorporated in this book.

Audience: Our audience for this book is intended to be diverse and includes clinicians, domain experts, clinical/financial analysts, managers, IT developers, consultants, vendors, policymakers, patients and consumers, executives, and lines-of-business leaders and researchers in academia. This book will find a home on the bookshelves of academic and industrial researchers and advanced students working in health care technology, biomedical engineering, and machine learning, thanks to contributions from a worldwide panel of renowned researchers. This edited book is appropriate for readers with no prior understanding of machine learning who want to implement machine-learning models in health care systems.

How Is This Book Organized? This book has ten chapters. Given our broad intended audience, it is put together in a way that appeals to different reader types and interests. While we strongly recommend reading the book sequentially, you have the flexibility to start with the chapters that interest you more than others.

Chapter 1 details the principles, challenges, and applications relating to internet of things (IoT) medical data analytics in health care. They touch on the viability of handling enormous volumes of heterogeneous data and of evidence-based decisions being taken to improve health care services. The tools and techniques used are also detailed. The chapter provides an overview of the data and knowledge discovery challenges associated with the field of health care informatics. It introduces the challenges of machine learning in the area and the relevant areas of investigation in the area.

Chapter 2 entails a system architecture of the internet of things (IoT) analysis of machine learning in health care systems. The role of artificial intelligence (AI) is unprecedented in this field. They discuss different AI classifiers for different dynamic areas and put forward a framework approach in addition to looking at data quality (as we do currently). The chapter also discusses how to use health care data analytics in current and next-generation analytics.

Chapter 3 gives a general overview of AI in health care with a special emphasis on brain-related disorders. AI in health care is expected to enable accurate diagnosis and fast service by gradually bringing efficient theoretical solutions to various brain-related disorders. The authors describe various deep learning approaches on the revelation of various neuroimaging disorders that display optimal performance even with large datasets.

Chapter 4 takes the insights of this book further by exploring the embedding of IoT in the Health care domain. Bibliometric analysis is done using Scopus and Web of Sciences datasets for IoT-enabled Health care applications using Machine Learning techniques. The study also demonstrates a "heart failure prediction" dataset for the study of machine learning algorithms in the IoT health care environment.

Chapter 5 focuses on smart health care technologies, which have given the health care business a new layer of "smartness." The chapter discusses in detail the wearable technology used to track user lifestyle choices and give tools for improved personal health management. Consider the most important AI and IoT applications in the field of health care. Furthermore, a variety of machine learning approaches have been elaborated to develop excellent decision support for health care applications.

Chapter 6 attempts to identify various health care data sources, characterize data, and explain the supervised machine learning detection models. An experimental study is put forward by using the decision tree classification technique for early prediction of polycystic ovarian syndrome. The results show 90% precision, and machine learning techniques predict the PCOS easily by taking some related factors into consideration. The results achieved will obviously be faster and more accurate than the manual doctor visits.

Chapter 7 discusses various wearable or implantable sensory devices used by individuals and the network architecture in a smart health care framework.

It also discusses the basics and underlying principles of the Internet of Medical Things (IoMT), Big Data, and ML techniques used in data-driven modern health care systems in detail. They also used different case studies, such as the health monitoring system, disease prediction, precision medicine, and clinical support system for better prediction of diseases, using machine learning methods to aid health care treatment techniques.

Chapter 8 lists the key objectives to understand the many data sources that influence a normal person's overall lifestyle (not having any specific severe disease). They have been successful in identifying those parameters and thorough understanding of the effects on lifestyle. Also, the study successfully integrated all the parameters into one system and provided a visualization in form of Azure TSI. Collecting more data from many users and constructing the first level of a generic model to predict lifestyle states for different age groups is one of the primary objectives of this work.

Chapter 9 discusses several perspectives on explainable artificial intelligence principles, as well as the understandability and interpretability of explainable AI systems, with a particular focus on the health care sector. This chapter uses AI explainability as a way to help build trustworthiness in the medical domain and takes a look at the recent developments in the area of explainable AI which encourages creativity, and at times are necessities in practice to raise awareness. The goal is to teach health care providers about the interpretability and understandability of explainable AI systems.

Chapter 10 investigates an empirical study of finding the automated classification techniques for classifying the sleep stages of subject-16 through C4-A1 channel. The study presented a novel comparison of channel effectiveness in the count to sleep scoring of sleep stages and the proposed method performed the best for scientific and clinical sleep disorder assessment.

Tawseef Ayoub Shaikh
Tabasum Rasool
Mohammed Wasid

Acknowledgment

We feel highly thankful to all the reviewers for their valuable feedback and evaluation of the chapters even in these tough times the world has met. A special thanks to the active research community, all public source databases and codes, and most importantly the SCI hub. Many authors have contributed to this book with their tremendous hard work and valuable time. We deeply thank them for their great contributions. In no particular order, they are: Akib Mohi Ud Din Khanday, Qamar Rayees Khan, Syed Tanzeel Rabani, Rumaan Bashir, Mahmood Hussain Mir, Dr Sanjay Jamwal, Shahidul Islam, Waseem Ahmad Mir, Dr Izharuddin, Junaid Ali Reshi, Ayushi Chahal, Preeti Gulia, Nasib Singh Gil, Dr. M. Deepika, Dr. D. Karthika, Anjume Shakir, E. Fantin Irudaya Raj, Nayana Gupta, N Manoj Kumar, Deepak Kumar Bagchi, Dr. Himani Mittal, Varun Srivastava, Shri Krishna Yadav, Suraj Kumar Prajapati, Dr Tawseef Ayoub Shaikh, Dr Tabasum Rasool, Abrar Rasool, Santosh Kumar Satapathy, Nakkala Srinivas Mudiraj, and Rupalin Nanda.

Chapter 1

Role of IoT in Smart Health Care Setups: A Critical Analysis

Akib Mohi Ud Din Khanday[1,*], Qamar Rayees Khan[2], Syed Tanzeel Rabani[1] and Rumaan Bashir[3]

[1]Research Lab, Department of Computer Sciences, BGSB University Rajouri, J&K, India

[2]Department of Computer Sciences, BGSB University, Rajouri, J&K, India

[3]Department of Computer Sciences, IUST, Awantipora, J&K, India

Abstract

The Internet of Things (IoT) has the potential to dramatically change how applications work in a variety of fields. The essential premise at the heart of this is that the IoT has the capability and amalgamation of various technologies to integrate both the physical and digital environments and ecosystems in a seamless manner. The Internet of Things (IoT) may be used in conjunction with real-time IT infrastructure to enjoy the advantages of connected objects and devices and create a seamless computing environment. Integration of the IoT into applications from a variety of different disciplines is possible. Healthcare, on the other hand, is one of the industries that has explicit opportunities to profit from the Internet of Things. Traditional healthcare services have been provided to patients since their origin, with current advancements including the introduction of IoT and digital technologies into the profession. A healthcare centre operates in a multipurpose manner in order to offer patients with the services they require. Physicians and medical professionals are working together to ensure that patients receive timely

[*]Corresponding Author's Email: akibkhanday@bgsbu.ac.in.

In: AI-Enabled IoT for Smart Health Care Systems
Editors: Tawseef Ayoub Shaikh, Tabasum Rasool and Mohammed Wasid
ISBN: 978-1-68507-977-2

treatment in order to avoid the occurrence of any unexpected medical conditions in the future. Today, it is critical to make use of available technology in order to improve the effectiveness and efficacy of medical aid, as well as to assist patients in improving their quality of life and their trust in the medical system, in order to achieve these goals. It also serves as a key to identifying current issues when the IoT is integrated into the healthcare system. In this chapter, a general overview of the IoT and its application areas in health care are examined in further depth.

Keywords: Internet of Things, healthcare, technologies, physicians

1. Introduction

Any healthcare facility's principal purpose is to give the highest quality of care and treatment to people who are in need of or require it. Healthcare that is dependable, accurate, and trustworthy is a fundamental demand for all human beings on the planet today. There is a tremendous impact on humankind as an outcome of the study being conducted in this field. During the current era of transformation from conventional healthcare to contemporary healthcare, numerous new technologies have emerged that are related to the improvement of Quality of Services (QoS) in the healthcare sector (Pederson and Leonard 2005; Khanday, Khan, and Rabani 2020b). These technologies include: Patients benefit from healthcare advances such as patient health monitoring devices and contemporary diagnostic equipment that is accurate and precise in its results. Healthcare applications that assist in the storage of patient data and the updating of that data on a regular basis as and when required. In order to provide patients with healthcare, healthcare centres have been utilising information and communication technology (also known as ICT) (Baraona et al. 2013). It has been stated that new innovations such as the IoT in healthcare. Implementation in healthcare can lead to exceptional and unparalleled levels of improvement in healthcare services if we keep the patient in mind as a receiver or consumer who need assistance. Specifically, this is the focus topic and hypothesis that has been used to build the basis for this study, which has as its purpose to analyse IoT applications in the healthcare domain in depth (Dlodlo, Mofolo, and Kagarura 2012).

Internet of Things offers opportunity to combine different technologies in order to create a more sophisticated network of things that enables connection between the real world and the digital interface. The benefits of being connected to a network and several technologies are inconceivable in today's world. Exemplifications of technologies RFID (also known as radio frequency identification) is a technology that allows physical things to be identified and interact with a digitally enabled environment, allowing them to be more productive. Implementation and realisation of the IoT bring intriguing and valuable applications while also posing significant problems.

2. IoT Set-Up Technologies

The following are the names of the technologies used for identification and tracking: Among the technologies that are being developed are "RFID," "EPC," "NFC," and "barcodes." They let individuals to engage with daily goods and services such as medical equipment and other gadgets, as well as link physical things to one another (Dlodlo, Mofolo, and Kagarura 2012). Physical objects may now be communicated with and interacted with thanks to ubiquitous WSNs, nanotechnology, embedded and linked tags and sensors, and other technologies. All of these wireless technologies have the capability of monitoring and collecting data about a variety of things, including tough to reach locations, the environment and wildlife as well as human vital signs. Wi-Fi, Bluetooth, and Zigbee are examples of previous communication technologies that have been brought together and linked to the internet or other network services. This is fundamental base for the IoT technology is to continue to develop and evolve in the future.

2.1. Sensors

The Internet of Things (IoT) includes a wide range of services and applications that are mostly reliant on sensors. The fundamental operations of applications are the monitoring and sensing of environmental variables, as well as the simple measurement of items through the use of sensors that are attached to them. It is the sensors, which are connected to the internet, that are responsible for this procedure. Sensing is a critical requirement for human-related applications since it allows the user to be interconnected with their environment in a smart way and feel the constantly changing ambient conditions. Sensors are small electrical devices that are a critical component of Internet of Things (IoT) technology. The sensors have the capability of sensing and measuring the ambient conditions of physical things such as temperature, air pressure, and pressure variations, among others. The sensors transform the observed value into either an analogue or a digitised representation, depending on the model. Using a communication channel, which can be wired or wirelessly connected, sensors can combine their data and send it to sensor nodes in a network. There are many different sensor types for a wide range of Internet of Things applications.

2.1.1. Temperature Sensor

This type of gadget is commonly found in all IoT-enabled environments, including agriculture, manufacturing, and the factory floor, where it is used to measure the temperature of the machine and track the temperature of the soil, among other things ("Top 15 Sensor Types Used By IoT Application Development Companies" n.d.).

2.1.2. Proximity Sensor

A gadget that detects the absence and presence of items in the immediate vicinity. These gadgets are most commonly found in retail environments. Proximity sensors can be used to monitor parking spaces, for example, parking space monitoring in a hospital or other facility (Lee and Lee 2015).

2.2. Wireless Sensor Networks

WSN is a critical component of the Internet of Things. When it comes to deploying IoT, wireless sensor network (WSN) technology is critical. WSN technology is a critical component of the Internet of Things since it consists of a collection of appropriate sensor nodes that are connected over the internet. They are responsible for tracking and monitoring the physical or environmental status, such as sound, temperature, and pressure, among other things. Sensor deployment with high-quality speed may be enabled by WSN technology, and the installation of a wireless sensor network can be completed in a matter of hours. WSNs are currently being employed in a variety of fields, including agriculture, the environment, industrial monitoring, and healthcare. WSNs are utilised in a wide range of surveillance and monitoring applications, and they are categorised as a type of mobile ad-hoc network (MANET) because of their mobility.

WSNs are most commonly employed in a variety of monitoring and surveillance applications, and they are classified as one of the mobile ad hoc network types, according to Wikipedia. Sensors are used to monitor and measure environmental parameters such as temperature, moisture fluctuations, the movement of animals in a certain region, rainfall, and other factors, among other things. The sensor node communicates with the main server by sending a site reference, which identifies the precise section where the modifications have occurred (Kuriakose, Amruth, and Nandhini 2014).Diverse applications enable the user to obtain information about the environment's condition (such as temperature) through the use of their smart phone, which may then be used to communicate with specific sensor nodes located in their region (Wang and Lin 2012).

2.3. Bluetooth

Bluetooth is a short-range wireless communication technology that allows data to be sent between devices over short distances and for the creation of personal area networks (PAN). Bluetooth technology enables short-range communication between small devices and other devices that are close by using radio waves. Class 1 Bluetooth has a range of up to 100 metres and class 2 Bluetooth has a range of 20 to 30 metres, depending on the model. Bluetooth smart is a new version of the Bluetooth technology that was introduced in 2012. It is a low-bandwidth, low-power, and low-cost wireless technology (Matsuoka et al. 2014), and it has the ability to deal with power consumption difficulties (Lin et al. 2014), making it a very good alternative for Internet of Things (IoT) implementation.

2.4. Barcode

The barcode is regarded as a significant invention that laid the groundwork for the development and expansion of RFID technology (Sörös 2014). An optical barcode is a specialised representation of data that is marked on everyday things such as bus tickets, train tickets, and other commercial products. It is readable by machines and can be read by humans. The barcode provides linked information about the things that carried the barcode, such as (product price and other connected information) about the objects that carried the barcode simply means that it recognises the physical objects (Z. Li and Chen 2014). Symbolic images consisting of combinations of bars with varied squares, dots, thickness, and other variety of forms in black and white and traceable by bar code reader (Grillo et al. 2010) are known as barcode images.

2.5. Radio Frequency Identification (RFID)

RFID is one of the most essential technologies of the Internet of Things since it makes use of radio waves to communicate between readers and tags (Duroc and Tedjini 2018). The primary goal of RFID is to discover and track physical items in order to monitor environmental factors through the use of tags that are connected to the objects themselves. In comparison to traditional RFID tags, RFID tags are smaller and comprise a small integrated circuit for the monitoring, storage, and processing of data. Additionally, tags modulate and demodulate the Radio Frequency signal are used. Active tags are powered by a battery and use radio waves to broadcast their signal. Passive tags do not require a power source and are therefore less expansive. However, they can remain alive and readable for an extended amount of time.

2.6. Wi-Fi

In the world of wireless networking, Wi-Fi is the name of a popular technology that makes use of radio waves to deliver high-speed internet and network connections ("Top 15 Sensor Types Used By IoT Application Development Companies" n.d.). Wi-Fi is an IEEE 802.11 base standard technology with a long range and a high transmission rate, and it is becoming increasingly popular. The technology of Wi-Fi is based on Wi-Fi is a wireless version of the ethernet network that was invented and made available by Wi-Fi Alliance (Coşkun, Ok, and Özdenizci Köse 2011). Nowadays, Wi-Fi can be used to link devices such as smartphones and tablets. Smart TVs, laptops, cameras, and printers that have the ability to connect to the internet are examples of such gadgets due to the fact that they are inside the range of any Wi-Fi network.

3. Related Work and Background

Internet of Things is evolved as a trending area for researchers to work on. The majority of work in IoT is related to Agriculture and Healthcare. In this section some of the notable research in the area of IoT is being discussed in detail.

3.1. Healthcare Information System Based on the IoT

The IoT technology, as well as its rapid advancements, assist in connecting smart items through the Internet in order to provide interoperable services in a distributed context. (Xu et al. 2014) presented insights on how the IoT is being used in healthcare, which has resulted in a massive increase in healthcare data. Data management and access methods to this massive amount of information are difficult to handle. Additionally, data in a variety of formats makes accessing the information more difficult. The Researchers are investigating the use of a resource-based data access mechanism known as UDA-IoT in the healthcare domain. They investigated the methods and ways of adopting an integrated approach in the healthcare information system so that data from multiple Internet of Things sources could be used. A semantic data paradigm for the storing and interpretation of Internet of Things data was proposed by the researchers. Interaction with the UDA-IoT is facilitated through fast delivery of data relevant to emergency medical services to all stakeholders. With the help of a case study known as emergency medical DSS, Xu and colleagues discussed their method (Decision Support System). The medical DSS is used to deal with medical emergencies that occur while using the DSS. In the implementation, "real-world entities," "alternative rescuing," "entity-oriented model," and "transition-oriented model" are included. There is also a persistence and execution engine, as well as cloud IoT data access services. Physicians and administrators in the healthcare system can use Internet of Things data sources to make well-informed judgments. (Rahmani et al. 2015) concentrated on gateways, which are used to bridge the gap between sensor networks and the Internet as part of the Internet of Things. They're utilised to provide services like "embedded data mining," "real-time local data processing," and "local storage" at a higher abstraction level. Furthermore, the gateway is capable of dealing with a wide range of difficulties, including "reliability," "scalability," and "energy efficiency." Using a proposed architecture, their study found that IoT-based health monitoring in hospitals may enhance "reliability," "security," "interoperability," "performance," and "energy efficiency," as well as increase patient safety and satisfaction. The IoT-driven smart architecture was proposed by (Catarinucci et al. 2015) as a tracking and monitoring media for automating the tracking and monitoring of people, medical equipment, and other things. According to the architecture guidelines, smart mobile, RFID, and WSN all play a critical role. Through the use of a virtual private network (VPN), secure remote access to healthcare infrastructure can be established.

(Gubbi et al. 2013) discussed the vision and future directions for the IoT. They offered a high-level overview of the Internet of Things, which is used for "sensing," "analytics," and "visualization" applications. (Oweis et al. 2016) also conducted research on similar applications of IoT. (Zhu et al. 2017) performed a case study to highlight the importance of the IoT. (Seo et al. 2016) presented an Internet of Things architecture that monitors food contamination, which is linked to concerns about human health. (Ganzha et al. 2017) investigated the semantic compatibility of different Internet of Things implementations. They also looked into the necessity of ontology in order to effectively implement IoT. Health ontologies, which provide the representation of healthcare knowledge, were described in detail by the authors. (Shah 2016) investigated how big data is constantly connected with the IoT, because the IoT generates a large amount of data that must be managed. Providing an overview of the IoT, (Y. Li et al. 2012) discussed how it is used for information exchange, assistance, and strategic decision making. (Danzl et al. 2016) investigated the requirement for quality of service and experience in rural health to reduce health concerns. The importance of education in the field of healthcare, as well as the development of technology that may be utilised to improve the overall quality of human life, were also highlighted.

(Santos et al. 2016) developed an m-Health scenario based on the IoT. An architecture based on mobile devices and healthcare infrastructure has been designed in order to construct an intelligent personal assistant (IPA). The widespread usage of mobile devices cleared the way for the implementation of IPA applications in the real world. These types of applications are primarily related with the healthcare industry. This method enables for the collecting of data on the patient's location, fall detection, heart rate, and other variables on an autonomous basis. (Tsai et al. 2016) explored metaheuristic algorithms in the context of healthcare, as well as the obstacles and issues associated with them. "Genetic algorithms" (GA), "particle swarm optimization" (PSO), "ant colony optimization" (ACO), and "support vector machines" (SVM) were investigated as algorithms that could be employed in healthcare systems, according to the researchers (Khanday, Khan, and Rabani, n.d., 2020a). They also presented a framework for big data analysis in the healthcare domain, which was well received. (Ahmed et al. 2015) stressed the necessity of teaching people about the Internet of Things. (Catarinucci et al. 2015) asserted that the number of wearable gadgets is expanding every single year. They are equipped with sensors to provide care to patients in healthcare facilities. In their report, they urged for the use of wearable gadgets in medical applications.

(Paschou et al. 2013) concentrated on the IoT in Healthcare (HIoT). Wearable devices, "heart rate monitors," "pulse oximeters," "glucose monitors," and "stethoscopes" are some of the associated technologies that have been identified for use in the implementation of IoT. All of these gadgets feature "Bluetooth," "Wi-Fi," and "RFID" integration capabilities. They also shared their insights on the expenses of data transfer associated with IoT integration in healthcare. They presented measurements for determining how effectively data is transferred.

(Ahmed et al. 2015) offered an overview of Internet of Things integration with health infrastructure for monitoring purposes. (Lee and Lee 2015) proposed that there are five critical technologies that are required in order to derive meaningful benefit from IoT adoption. RFID, IoT middleware, IoT application software, WSN, and cloud computing are some of the technologies involved.

3.2. RFID, EPC, and Barcode's Role in IoT-Based Healthcare Units

Using RFID technology and an RFID reader, (Rahmani et al. 2015) looked at whether RFID technology and an RFID reader are important in the hardware abstraction of smart e-health gateways. RFID, according to (Catarinucci et al. 2015), low-power, low-cost technology that uses tags to participate in calculations by transmitting data to RFID readers. RFID tags are small devices that transmit data to RFID readers. RFID tags do not waste energy and have a lifespan of several decades, which makes the technology suited for Internet of Things applications. The Ultra-High-Frequency (UHF) RFID technology is a variation on the RFID technology that has extra capabilities, including the ability to sense and compute. In healthcare institutions, the increased use of mobile devices paved the path for the real-world deployment of IPA apps. RFID tags have the potential to integrate sensing and computational functions. RFID tags operate within the range of the reader's coverage. The application of RFID technology is limited to the monitoring of patients or medical devices. (Madanian 2016) investigated e-Health technology and shed light on RFID technology, among other things. They believe that RFID will play a significant role in the realisation of the IoT and its connection with healthcare infrastructure. RFID is, in fact, required for the identification of medical equipment and any other physical object that want to engage in computers. A large number of components are required for an RFID system. An antenna, an

RFID reader with an RF module, an RFID tag, and a host computer or device are all included.

3.3. Internet of Things Wearables

The IoT can bring the physical and digital worlds together. Wearable IoT is a new version of the IoT that has developed as a result of the advent of wearable devices in the healthcare industry (WIoT). This kind of network may help healthcare professionals monitor individual health information so that they can offer tailored wellness and health services to people who need them. (Hiremath, Yang, and Mankodiya 2014) proposed an Internet of Things architecture. There are three major components that make up the Internet of Things. "Wearable body area sensors," "Internet-connected gateways," support for "cloud and big data," and other related technologies are among them. A wireless connection connects body-worn devices to medical infrastructure. "Therapeutic sensors," "onbody contact sensors," "health and wellness sensors," "behavioural sensors," and "rehabilitation sensors" are some of the types of body area sensors that are currently available. Sensors for rehabilitation help with language development and assistive technologies for the blind. Sensors are used to measure falls, sleeping patterns, and exercise, as well as emotions like worry, sadness, and tension, and nutrition like eating habits and calorie intake. In addition to tracking mobility, calorie count and physical activity, fitness and wellness sensors also track location information, such as GPS information and indoor localisation. Drug delivery sensors, stimulation sensors for chronic pain management, and emergency sensors for defibrillators are all examples of therapeutic sensors in the medical field. Monitoring sensors detect physiological signals like ECG, EMG, and EEG, as well as chemical signals like saliva, glucose, and perspiration, and visual signals like tissue characteristics and oximetry. Physiological signals such as ECG, EMG, and EEG are also detected by monitoring devices. In the future, personalised healthcare services will play an essential role. Personalized health services in smart homes were discussed by (Datta et al. 2015), who shed light on the possibility of such services. In order to provide tailored healthcare services, they presented an architectural solution. Sensor devices, an M2K gateway, networking technologies, cloud storage, and access control methods are all part of the architecture.

3.4. Internet of Things for Telehealth at Home

In the context of healthcare, the practise of using telecommunication technology by patients and healthcare service providers to guarantee an equal flow of information about healthcare is known as home telehealth. (Chen and Hsiao 2012) investigated the possibility of using the Internet of Things to implement home telehealth. They demonstrated a technology called CogSense, which was designed to facilitate real-time healthcare services by bringing together patients, clinicians, and caregivers in a collaborative and coordinated effort. Their system includes sensors that monitor patients' health, as well as communication technologies and data analysis that may be utilised to make better choices. It is feasible to have realisable services with tailored data storage and retrieval by using a cloud-enabled method to data storage and retrieval.

4. Impact of IoT on Healthcare

The provision of healthcare services and the availability of a medical information system are nearly connected with national welfare and the standard of life (Pederson and Leonard 2005). The IoT has the potential to provide number of healthcare applications, including chronic diseases, remote monitoring, senior care, and exercise programmes. Another noteworthy possible use is the provision of compliance and medical care at home through smart healthcare services. In this manner, "medical devices," "Imaging," and "diagnostic" equipment may all be regarded as smart devices that are part of Internet of Things system. Healthcare services based on the IoT improve quality of life while simultaneously reducing treatment costs and enhancing the user experience (Ghoshdastider, Viga, and Kraft 2014). The IoT is essential for staying safe, increasing efficiency, and improving overall healthcare monitoring and management quality. The IoT encompasses important technologies like RFID and smart sensors, which may enable health data transfer, smart health monitoring, and precise location (Sun et al. 2012; Medaglia and Serbanati 2010). Hospitals can also benefit from the Internet of Things by streamlining tracking administration and patient monitoring (Prasad and Reichert 2011; Khanday et al. 2020). When it comes to IoT, networks are networks that communicate and connect physical objects, which are then converted into digital things by utilising the internet and communication channels [9]. These infrastructures are made up of existing and connecting

Internet connections, as well as network expansion. A specific object identification system, sensors, and association capability will be offered as the starting point for the advancement of autonomous supportive services and the development of apps. These will be differentiated by the large amount of data storage, data transport, network affiliation, and interoperability that they offer to users. Nowadays, the IoT connects sensors and a plethora of devices, with the majority of them communicating via IP-based communications. IoT currently links with smart sensors and a huge number of medical equipment through the use of Internet protocol-based communication networks.

In the healthcare industry, the IoT provides patients with services such as remote monitoring, early diagnosis, and prevention. In the Internet of Things, patients can be hooked to or implanted with actuators, sensors, and RFID tags, among other things. These gadgets and accompanying tags provide patients' information to family members, physicians, and nurses, among other people. These RFID tags attached to medical devices that are attached to patients are identifiable, controlled, readable, and traceable through the IoT application (Tesoriero et al. 2009). The IoT enables a variety of services and smart applications to address the issues that the healthcare industry faces (Medaglia and Serbanati 2010). The IoT has the potential to connect patients and doctors, devices and machines, patients and machines, sensors and mobile devices, tags and readers, and mobile devices and humans. A healthcare system that is efficient is provided by intelligently connecting machines, humans, smart devices, and systems (Yang et al. 2012). The following are examples of IoT applications in real life. The IoT has a plethora of health-care applications, such as a wearable hospital staff support system that can be used to locate both patients and physicians in the hospital at any time. More applications, such as an Internet of Things information system, can be added to discover any adverse drug reactions in patients. The combination of "smart sensors," "innovative technologies," and "Wi-Fi" proves to be quite beneficial in the monitoring of vital signs such as "blood pressure," "cholesterol levels," "temperature," and "heart rate," among others. Body-worn sensors that are implanted in patients with chronic diseases collect and store information about their health. By monitoring chronic disease and medication management using ambient and wearable sensors, there are a number of Internet of Things applications which have a significant impact on ageing people's ability to live independently (Dlodlo, Mofolo, and Kagarura 2012).

5. IoT's Potential Application in Healthcare

When the Internet of Things is coupled with health infrastructure, healthcare units can have a variety of apps that can serve patients in an attractive manner. According to (Dlodlo, Mofolo, and Kagarura 2012), "Diabetes management," "cardiovascular disease management," "environmental health," "occupational health," "nutrition," "mental health," "home and community-based healthcare," "emergency services," "sports and fitness," "Infant care," "oral health," "disease surveillance," "telemedicine," "chronic medical management," and "ambient assisted living for the elderly" are just a few of the applications available. Figure 1. Depicts the various applications of IoT in Healthcare.

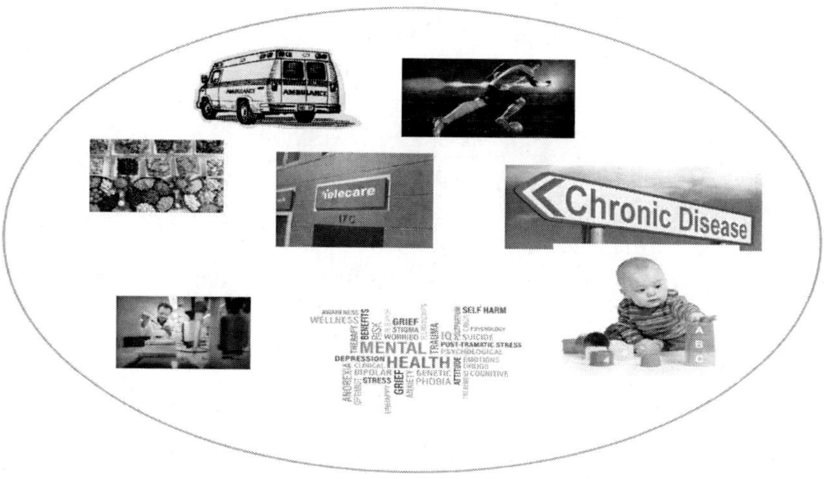

Figure 1. Application areas of IoT in Healthcare.

5.1. Living with the Help of the Environment

As a result of higher life expectancy, there are more elderly people in many countries. They require extra attention during their adult years in order to live a self-sufficient and independent existence. The Internet of Things technology deployed in healthcare institutions can provide ambient-assisted living. The Internet of Things, in conjunction with healthcare infrastructure, provides particular services to the elderly, which can improve the overall quality of life for adults. One of the platforms for ambient assisted living that is now accessible is

Caalyx-MV. It is designed to provide healthcare services to the general adult population, as well as to children. In order to accomplish this, the home system makes use of a variety of gadgets that perform computations. The ambient-assisted living platform includes a variety of devices and aspects that are designed specifically for elderly persons. The services are obtained with the assistance of the Internet (Dlodlo, Mofolo, and Kagarura 2012). Another system that contributes to the success of ambient-assisted living is confidence. It made use of radio tags that were attached to the body. The system has the capability of monitoring patients, reconstructing their posture, and detecting any irregularities. It is capable of detecting falls and being left unattended. Elderly persons can live confidently and comfortably if they have confidence in their abilities (Luštrek, Gams, and Vélez 2009).

5.2. Medication Treatment for Chronic Conditions

Patients with chronic illnesses must adhere to their treatment regimen for an extended period of time (Baraona et al. 2013). In this case, a patient's failure to comply can have devastating repercussions for him or her. It also has the additional effect of raising the expense of further healthcare services and medications. Chronic medicine can be tracked with the help of Internet of Things integration. It is feasible to link RFID tags to medical devices in order to track the devices' movements. In this instance, automatic information acquisition is accomplished through the use of RFID and EPC. It is feasible to assist patients with chronic diseases in receiving the most appropriate medication as prescribed by their physicians through the use of these technologies as part of the Internet of Things. The visualisation and monitoring of the pharmaceutical supply chain can aid in the improvement of the quality of services connected to chronic medication management (Dlodlo, Mofolo, and Kagarura 2012). Correctospecto and the Philips medication dispensing service are only a couple of the services that are available in this area (Oweis et al. 2016).

5.3. Tele-Care

According to the World Health Organization (Organization 2010), Telemedicine is a term that refers to the provision of medical treatment through audiovisual conversations and data exchanges, which includes diagnosing and treating medical problems, educating patients, transmitting medical data, and diagnosing and treating diseases. Telemedicine services are provided by a variety of divisions within healthcare organisations. Patients who are at home usually communicate with one another via the Internet. These calls are answered by representatives from service providers. Then service providers take the initiative to bring in a qualified doctor to assist them in comprehending, diagnosing, and resolving their patients' problems. Voice-based communication is the main method of communication. This type of application allows patients to communicate with care providers and receive professional guidance without having to leave their homes. In addition to saving time and money, this can boost their morale and confidence in their abilities.

5.4. Disease Monitoring

Disease surveillance can aid in the development of more effective tactics for combating disease outbreaks (Rabani, Khan, and Khanday 2020). Disease surveillance can be carried out by healthcare organisations and governments with the help of IoT-enabled healthcare services. Google Flu Trends is a web-based programme developed by Google that tracks online behaviour and keeps track of influenza outbreaks. If you compare Twitter's ability to identify cholera epidemics with that of healthcare professionals, you'll see that Twitter is just as effective. An programme called Health map gives users the ability to keep track of worldwide trends in disease outbreaks (Hiremath, Yang, and Mankodiya 2014). It provides consumers with timely notifications about various ailments and the severity of such conditions. These types of services can be provided in real time through the use of Internet of Things integration, hence improving accuracy and quality. The Health Map application takes use of technologies, "geospatial information systems," "global positioning systems," and "radio frequency identification" are just a few examples.

5.5. Managing Oral Health

This is connected to oral health, which includes dental problems, among other things. Due to the association that exists between diseases such as diabetes, respiratory sickness, cardiovascular disease, and issues of pregnancy, preventive dental care is absolutely necessary. Oral health management has grown easier as a result of technological advancements and Internet of Things integration with healthcare infrastructure (Dlodlo, Mofolo, and Kagarura 2012).

5.6. Child Care

As a child grows into an adult, infant care becomes increasingly crucial in any community. It is necessary to make efforts to safeguard babies from diseases. "Immunization" and "vaccination" are critical for the prevention and treatment of a variety of diseases, including measles, "TB," and "polio." RFID tags and sensors can aid in the improvement of the overall quality of baby care. In order to provide real-time care for babies, it is critical to maintain track of their body temperature and other vital signs. This is made possible by the IoT, which is employed in healthcare units (Dlodlo, Mofolo, and Kagarura 2012).

5.7. Health and Lifestyle

With IoT enabling healthcare services, it is feasible to monitor health and lifestyle. As discussed in (Shah 2016; Dlodlo, Mofolo, and Kagarura 2012), athletes may benefit from mobile apps linked with sensors that track their activity. Not only can the programmes maintain track of activities, but they can also keep track of things like "time spent," "speed," and so on. In addition, it integrates with Google Maps to provide navigation. Sports fitness activities can be recorded using CardioTrainer, another application that works on Android smart phones and uses GPS tracking to track the progress of athletes. When athletes use Internet of Things-related gadgets and applications, they are reminded about time, cycles, and other important information through real-time voice messages.

5.8. First-Aid Services

Medical treatments are frequently delayed as a result of the distance between the healthcare facility and the patient's residence. There is a significant lag in getting to the hospital. Furthermore, both money and time are at stake. A similar situation can arise in an emergency situation as well, unless an alternate plan is put in place. In order to overcome this challenge, IoT applications related with healthcare can be modified in order to conduct real-time observations of patients, whether they are at home or on the road. Even before a patient arrives at the hospital, it is possible to begin treating him or her. The mobile nodes included in the Internet of Things, sensor devices, and healthcare infrastructure all collaborate to ensure real-time communication among the various parties involved. Real-time delivery of patient vital signs is made feasible by the use of machine-to-machine interaction. This has a significant impact on the delivery of healthcare services (Dlodlo, Mofolo, and Kagarura 2012).

5.9. Community-Based and Health-Centered Care

People who are associated with communities have a higher quality of life as a result of community-based healthcare services. When patients are not recommended to relocate for any reason, these services are offered in the comfort of their own homes. Patients with physical disabilities and those suffering from chronic ailments, for example, can benefit from such services. With the development of technologies and the use of NFS-enabled devices, an intuitive interface between devices and patients has been created (Dlodlo, Mofolo, and Kagarura 2012). When examining RFID compatibility with NFS, it becomes clear that these technologies can be beneficial in providing improved healthcare services.

5.10. Mental Health

Unfortunately, mental health is frequently neglected. It can be inferred in the aforementioned case because it is disregarded without a diagnosis (Rabani, Rayees Khan, and Khanday 2020). The integration of IoT applications with healthcare, as demonstrated in (Dlodlo, Mofolo, and Kagarura 2012), can help to reduce this problem. Individuals suffering from some mental health illnesses, such as Generalized Anxiety Disorder (GAD), may experience long-term consequences. Treatment of such disorders necessitates the use of behavioural, cognitive, and physical methods. Biofeedback, making patients aware of their own reactions to situations, as well as teaching them through various programmes, all help to reduce the severity of the illness.

5.11. Nutrition

The importance of nutrition in healthcare services cannot be overstated. When it is ignored, it can lead to a variety of health problems. The Internet of Things (IoT) in conjunction with healthcare units can provide education and timely counselling to ensure that people's dietary concerns are properly addressed. It is possible to solve nutrition-based allergies and their associated side effects by utilising IoT applications linked with healthcare infrastructure and wearable devices worn by patients (Dlodlo, Mofolo, and Kagarura 2012).

Conclusion

In today's high-tech world, the IoT has emerged as a true trailblazer and game changer in the effort to provide patients with incredibly high-quality healthcare services. There is a plethora of technologies and applications available on the Internet that provide remarkable opportunities for physicians and experts to analyse patient information, track and monitor patients' health in an optimised and highly productive manner, allowing them to recommend highly reliable medication and treatment to their patients. The Internet of Things (IoT) definitions, concept, and role in healthcare services have all been explored in this chapter. Sensors, WSN, NFC, barcode, RFID, and other IoT-enabled technologies have also been discussed in the chapter, for example. The IoT-based information system for healthcare services has been investigated. IoT applications in a variety of healthcare fields have been presented, along with insights into how IoT technologies are providing the required architecture and system to improve the quality of healthcare services. The benefits of the IoT have been studied in a variety of healthcare settings, including emergency situations.

References

Ahmed, Mobyen Uddin, Mats Björkman, Aida Čaušević, Hossein Fotouhi, and Maria Lindén. 2015. "An Overview on the Internet of Things for Health Monitoring Systems." In *International Internet of Things Summit*, 429–36. Springer.

Baraona, Fernando, Michelle Gurvitz, Michael J Landzberg, and Alexander R Opotowsky. 2013. "Hospitalizations and Mortality in the United States for Adults With Down Syndrome and Congenital Heart Disease." *The American Journal of Cardiology* 111 (7): 1046–51. https://doi.org/https://doi.org/10.1016/j.amjcard.2012.12.025.

Catarinucci, Luca, Danilo De Donno, Luca Mainetti, Luca Palano, Luigi Patrono, Maria Laura Stefanizzi, and Luciano Tarricone. 2015. "An IoT-Aware Architecture for Smart Healthcare Systems." *IEEE Internet of Things Journal* 2 (6): 515–26.

Chen, Rai-Fu, and Ju-Ling Hsiao. 2012. "An Investigation on Physicians' Acceptance of Hospital Information Systems: A Case Study." *International Journal of Medical Informatics* 81 (12): 810–20.

Coşkun, Vedat, Kerem Ok, and Büşra Özdenizci Köse. 2011. "Near Field Communication: From Theory to Practice." John Wiley and Sons.

Danzl, Megan M, Anne Harrison, Elizabeth G Hunter, Janice Kuperstein, Violet Sylvia, Katherine Maddy, and Sarah Campbell. 2016. "'A Lot of Things Passed Me by': Rural Stroke Survivors' and Caregivers' Experience of Receiving Education From Health Care Providers." *The Journal of Rural Health* 32 (1): 13–24. /https://doi.org/10.1111/jrh.12124.

Datta, SK, C Bonnet, A Gyrard, RP Ferreira da Costa, and K Boudaoud. 2015. "Applying Internet of Things for Personalized Healthcare in Smart Homes." In *2015 24th Wireless and Optical Communication Conference (WOCC)*, 164–69. https://doi.org/10.1109/WOCC.2015.7346198.

Dlodlo, Nomusa, Mofolo Mofolo, and Geoffrey Mark Kagarura. 2012. "Potential Applications of the Internet of Things in Sustainable Rural Development in South Africa." *Adv. Inf. Technol. Appl. Comput.* 1 (August): 180–88.

Duroc, Yvan, and Smail Tedjini. 2018. "RFID: A Key Technology for Humanity." *Comptes Rendus Physique* 19 (1–2): 64–71.

Ganzha, Maria, Marcin Paprzycki, Wiesław Pawłowski, Paweł Szmeja, and Katarzyna Wasielewska. 2017. "Semantic Interoperability in the Internet of Things: An Overview from the INTER-IoT Perspective." *Journal of Network and Computer Applications* 81: 111–24.

Ghoshdastider, Unmesh, Reinhard Viga, and Michael Kraft. 2014. "Non-Invasive Synchronized Spatially High-Resolution Wireless Body Area Network." In *2014 IEEE Ninth International Conference on Intelligent Sensors, Sensor Networks and Information Processing (ISSNIP)*, 1–6. IEEE.

Grillo, Antonio, Alessandro Lentini, Marco Querini, and Giuseppe F Italiano. 2010. "High Capacity Colored Two Dimensional Codes." In *Proceedings of the International Multiconference on Computer Science and Information Technology*, 709–16. IEEE.

Gubbi, Jayavardhana, Rajkumar Buyya, Slaven Marusic, and Marimuthu Palaniswami. 2013. "Internet of Things (IoT): A Vision, Architectural Elements, and Future Directions." *Future Generation Computer Systems* 29 (7): 1645–60.

Hiremath, Shivayogi, Geng Yang, and Kunal Mankodiya. 2014. "Wearable Internet of Things: Concept, Architectural Components and Promises for Person-Centered Healthcare." In *2014 4th International Conference on Wireless Mobile Communication and Healthcare-Transforming Healthcare Through Innovations in Mobile and Wireless Technologies (MOBIHEALTH)*, 304–7. IEEE.

Khanday, Akib Mohi Ud Din, Qamar Rayees Khan, and Syed Tanzeel Rabani. n.d. "SVMBPI : Support Vector Machine Based Propaganda Identification ."

———. 2020a. "Detecting Textual Propaganda Using Machine Learning Techniques." *Baghdad Science Journal*, no. December: 199–209. https://doi.org/http://dx.doi.org/10.21123/bsj.2020.18.1.5251.

———. 2020b. "Identifying Propaganda from Online Social Networks during COVID-19 Using Machine Learning Techniques." *International Journal of Information Technology*. https://doi.org/10.1007/s41870-020-00550-5.

Khanday, Akib Mohi Ud Din, Syed Tanzeel Rabani, Qamar Rayees Khan, Nusrat Rouf, and Masarat Mohi ud Din. 2020. "Machine Learning Based Approaches for Detecting COVID-19 Using Clinical Text Data." *International Journal of Information Technology*. https://doi.org/10.1007/s41870-020-00495-9.

Kuriakose, Jeril, V Amruth, and N Swathy Nandhini. 2014. "A Survey on Localization of Wireless Sensor Nodes." In *International Conference on Information Communication and Embedded Systems (ICICES2014)*, 1–6. IEEE.

Lee, In, and Kyoochun Lee. 2015. "The Internet of Things (IoT): Applications, Investments, and Challenges for Enterprises." *Business Horizons* 58 (4): 431–40.

Li, Yuan, Mingjun Hou, Heng Liu, and Yi Liu. 2012. "Towards a Theoretical Framework of Strategic Decision, Supporting Capability and Information Sharing under the Context of Internet of Things." *Information Technology and Management* 13 (4): 205–16.

Li, Zhigang, and Weiwei Chen. 2014. "D&S Barcode: A Dynamic and Sensitive Barcode for Intelligent Environment Monitoring." In *2014 International Conference on Intelligent Environments*, 47–51. IEEE.

Lin, Zhe-Min, Cheng-Hung Chang, Nai-Kuan Chou, and Yuan-Hsiang Lin. 2014. "Bluetooth Low Energy (BLE) Based Blood Pressure Monitoring System." In *2014 International Conference on Intelligent Green Building and Smart Grid (IGBSG)*, 1–4. IEEE.

Luštrek, Mitja, Matjaž Gams, and Igone Vélez. 2009. "Posture and Movement Monitoring for Ambient Assisted Living." IST-Africa.

Madanian, Samaneh. 2016. "The Use of E-Health Technology in Healthcare Environment: The Role of RFID Technology." In *2016 10th International Conference on E-Commerce in Developing Countries: With Focus on e-Tourism (ECDC)*, 1–5. IEEE.

Matsuoka, Hideki, Junbo Wang, Lei Jing, Yinghui Zhou, Yilang Wu, and Zixue Cheng. 2014. "Development of a Control System for Home Appliances Based on BLE Technique." In *2014 IEEE International Symposium on Independent Computing (ISIC)*, 1–5. IEEE.

Medaglia, Carlo Maria, and Alexandru Serbanati. 2010. "An Overview of Privacy and Security Issues in the Internet of Things." *The Internet of Things*, 389–95.

Organization, World Health. 2010. *Telemedicine: Opportunities and Developments in Member States. Report on the Second Global Survey on EHealth.* World Health Organization.

Oweis, Nour E, Claudio Aracenay, Waseem George, Mona Oweis, Hussein Soori, and Vaclav Snasel. 2016. "Internet of Things: Overview, Sources, Applications and Challenges." In *Proceedings of the Second International Afro-European Conference for Industrial Advancement AECIA 2015*, 57–67. Springer.

Paschou, Mersini, Evangelos Sakkopoulos, Efrosini Sourla, and Athanasios Tsakalidis. 2013. "Health Internet of Things: Metrics and Methods for Efficient Data Transfer." *Simulation Modelling Practice and Theory* 34: 186–99.

Pederson, Lorraine, and Kevin Leonard. 2005. "Measuring Information Technology Investment among Canadian Academic Health Sciences Centres." *Healthcare Quarterly (Toronto, Ont.)* 8 (1): 94–101; discussion 102. http://europepmc.org/abstract/MED/15715341.

Prasad, Ramjee, and Frank Reichert. 2011. "Special Issue on 'Internet of Things and Future Applications.'" *Wireless Personal Communications* 61 (3): 491–93.

Rabani, Syed Tanzeel, Qamar Rayees Khan, and Akib Mohi Ud Din Khanday. 2020. "Detection of Suicidal Ideation on Twitter Using Machine Learning & Ensemble Approaches." *Baghdad Science Journal* 17 (4): 1328–39. https://doi.org/10.21123/bsj.2020.17.4.1328.

Rabani, Syed Tanzeel, Qamar Rayees Khan, and Akib Mohi Ud Din Khanday. 2020. "Multi-Class Suicide Risk Prediction on Twitter Using Machine Learning Techniques." In *2020 2nd International Conference on Advances in Computing, Communication Control and Networking (ICACCCN)*, 128–34. https://doi.org/10.1109/ICACCCN51052.2020.9362979.

Rahmani, Amir-Mohammad, Nanda Kumar Thanigaivelan, Tuan Nguyen Gia, Jose Granados, Behailu Negash, Pasi Liljeberg, and Hannu Tenhunen. 2015. "Smart E-Health Gateway: Bringing Intelligence to Internet-of-Things Based Ubiquitous Healthcare Systems." In *2015 12th Annual IEEE Consumer Communications and Networking Conference (CCNC)*, 826–34. IEEE.

Santos, João, Joel JPC Rodrigues, Bruno MC Silva, João Casal, Kashif Saleem, and Victor Denisov. 2016. "An IoT-Based Mobile Gateway for Intelligent Personal Assistants on Mobile Health Environments." *Journal of Network and Computer Applications* 71: 194–204.

Seo, Sung-Min, Seung-Wan Kim, Jin-Woo Jeon, Jee-Hyun Kim, Hee-Soo Kim, Jung-Hwan Cho, Won-Ho Lee, and Se-Hwan Paek. 2016. "Food Contamination Monitoring via Internet of Things, Exemplified by Using Pocket-Sized Immunosensor as Terminal Unit." *Sensors and Actuators B: Chemical* 233: 148–56.

Shah, Mohak. 2016. "Big Data and the Internet of Things." In *Big Data Analysis: New Algorithms for a New Society*, 207–37. Springer.

Sörös, Gábor. 2014. "GPU-Accelerated Joint 1D and 2D Barcode Localization on Smartphones." In *2014 IEEE International Conference on Acoustics, Speech and Signal Processing (ICASSP)*, 5095–99. IEEE.

Sun, Qingfeng, Fansen Kong, Ling Zhang, and Xiangwen Dang. 2012. "Construction of Emergency Evacuation Information System Based on the Internet of Things." *International Information Institute (Tokyo). Information* 15 (12): 5363.

Tesoriero, Ricardo, José A Gallud, María D Lozano, and Víctor M R Penichet. 2009. "Tracking Autonomous Entities Using RFID Technology." *IEEE Transactions on Consumer Electronics* 55 (2): 650–55.

"Top 15 Sensor Types Used By IoT Application Development Companies." n.d. Accessed February 12, 2022. https://www.finoit.com/blog/top-15-sensor-types-used-iot/.

Tsai, Chun-Wei, Ming-Chao Chiang, Adlen Ksentini, and Min Chen. 2016. "Metaheuristic Algorithms for Healthcare: Open Issues and Challenges." *Computers & Electrical Engineering* 53: 421–34.

Wang, Jing, and Xiaola Lin. 2012. "User Dispersed Authentication Scheme for Wireless Sensor Networks." In *2012 Fourth International Conference on Digital Home*, 411–14. IEEE.

Xu, Boyi, Li Da Xu, Hongming Cai, Cheng Xie, Jingyuan Hu, and Fenglin Bu. 2014. "Ubiquitous Data Accessing Method in IoT-Based Information System for Emergency Medical Services." *IEEE Transactions on Industrial Informatics* 10 (2): 1578–86.

Yang, Po, Wenyan Wu, Mansour Moniri, and Claude C Chibelushi. 2012. "Efficient Object Localization Using Sparsely Distributed Passive RFID Tags." *IEEE Transactions on Industrial Electronics* 60 (12): 5914–24.

Zhu, Tao, Sahraoui Dhelim, Zhihao Zhou, Shunkun Yang, and Huansheng Ning. 2017. "An Architecture for Aggregating Information from Distributed Data Nodes for Industrial Internet of Things." *Computers & Electrical Engineering* 58: 337–49.

Chapter 2

Internet of Things in Health Care: Architecture, Technologies, Protocols, Applications, Challenges and Future Scope

Mahmood Hussain Mir*, **Sanjay Jamwal and Shahidul Islam**

Department of Computer Sciences, Baba Ghulam Shah Badshah University, Rajouri, Jammu & Kashmir, India-185234

Abstract

Internet of Things is a recent and promising area of mobile and pervasive computing; mobility and pervasiveness are the two most important characteristics of a mobile and pervasive communication system. In technical terms, the Internet of Things can be referred as the Internet of Objects, or Object-Oriented Internetworking (OOI). It focuses on the fact that objects are connected over the Internet rather than people. IoT is an internetworking of daily objects with some sort of intelligence. IoT is opening vast opportunities for many new applications areas that will change the livelihood of the people. During the last decade, IoT is attracting more curiosity from researchers and industrialists around the globe. Internet of Things is made up of two terms, Internet and Things. Things refer to physical objects with any inbuilt communication technology such as Infrared, RFID, Bluetooth and Wi-Fi, etc. The Internet refers to the internetworking of objects through which objects are communicating with each other. This survey aims to come up with an extensive survey on the main components such as architecture, enabling technologies and protocols, and applications of IoT. This survey is

*Corresponding Author's Email: mahmoodhussain@bgsbu.ac.in.

In: AI-Enabled IoT for Smart Health Care Systems
Editors: Tawseef Ayoub Shaikh, Tabasum Rasool and Mohammed Wasid
ISBN: 978-1-68507-977-2

dedicated to those who want to add to the development of this novel field in such a ubiquitous scenario. Furthermore, some challenges, issues, and future scope are also discussed.

Keywords: IoT, protocol, RFID, sensor, WSN, actuator, transducer

1. Introduction

The Internet of Things (IoT) is a situation in which network communication and processing capabilities extend beyond computers to smart devices such as objects, sensors, and even everyday objects, allowing them to generate, share, and consume data with little or no human engagement (Atzori, Iera, and Morabito 2010). Peter Lewis coined the phrase "Internet of Things" in November 1985 at a US Commerce Department conference (Ladd and Groth 2015). Following the conference, the term "internet of things" became widespread in the late 1990s. Kevin Ashton of Proctor and Gamble (P&G) mentioned the Internet of Things later in his 1999 presentation (Pfeifer 2012). He then co-founded the Auto-ID Centre at the Massachusetts Institute of Technology (MIT). Ashton produced an article for the RFID Journal in 2009 in which he addressed the Internet of Things in great detail (Ray 2018). IoT was included in Ashton's inventory management systems (RFID devices). There is no globally agreed definition for the "Internet of Things," which is a worldwide term that requires a common meaning. The ITU-T IoT-GSI (IoT Global Standards Initiative) team has described the Internet of Things as follows: "*A global infrastructure for the information society that enables improved services through the interconnection of (physical and virtual) things based on existing and evolving interoperable information and communication technologies*" (Of and Cities 2018). "*A dynamic global network infrastructure with self-configuring capabilities based on standard and interoperable communication protocols where physical and virtual things have identities, physical attributes, and virtual personalities, use intelligent interfaces and are seamlessly integrated into the information network*", according to the IERC definition (Vermesan, O., Friess, P., Guillemin, P., Gusmeroli, S., n.d.).

The ITU and IERC define the IoT as a dynamic and global network architecture with self-configuring capability based on industry standards Communication Technologies and Protocols (CERP-IOT 2008). Architecture, transducer (sensor/actuator), connectivity, identification (addressing), and other technologies are all used in IoT. The IoT is based on the ubiquitous presence of many things or products that use a Radio Access Network (RAN) such as Bluetooth, ZigBee, or Wi-Fi with RFID tags (Bhuvaneswari and Porkodi 2014). RFID tags have a unique identification (address) that enables products or things to interact and collaborate towards a common goal.

In 2011, the number of Internet of Things devices overtook the number of people on the globe, and by 2025, it is projected that the number of IoT devices will be between 30 billion and 50 billion. There will be over five more types of devices having native Internet access (Ivanov 2014).

According to IDC, by 2025, the IoT market will have grown to 300 billion devices, with 30 billion of them being connected. According to IDC, the installed sophisticated solutions that collect data across consumer and business applications will drive this expansion ("IoT End-User Perceptions, Strategies and Preferences in Hungary" 2018).

The IoT is a worldwide network that allows humans, things, and things-to-things to communicate with one another, as well as anything else in the world, by assigning each object a unique identity (Madakam, Ramaswamy, and Tripathi 2015). "Device-to-device", "device-to-cloud", and "device-to-gateway" are all terms that can apply to anybody, everywhere, at any time. The IoT scenario is depicted in Figure 1.

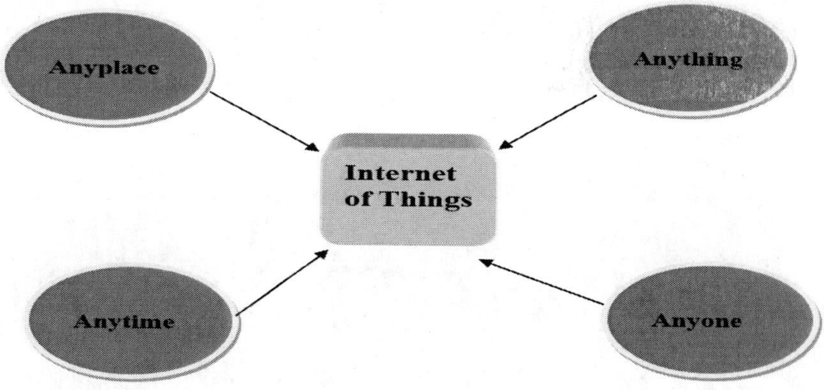

Figure 1. Scenario of IoT.

2. General Architecture

Because the IoT is a new concept, no standard architecture has been established by organizations such as IEEE, ITU-T, ETSI, IETF, CEN/ISO,

GSI, and others. A layered architecture is the focus of both researchers and industrialists. IoT is made up of three layers when seen in a layered approach (Lin et al. 2017). The majority of the IoT work is based on wireless sensor networks. The layered architecture is divided into two sections, each with a network or transport layer that serves as a common communication medium. The sensing layer is meant for data capture, while the application layer is responsible for data consumption in applications (Singh and Singh Tomar 2019).

Nowadays, the internet and the actual world are separated, and communication between them is primarily based on human-computer interaction. In the actual world, some apps automatically monitor or manipulate environment items in an intelligent manner (Islam et al. 2015). These intelligent applications can be considered the first IoT application attempt. The "internet of things", the "internet of services", and the "internet of networks" are all crucial characteristics of the future IoT. Every object in nature is connected to or observed by ubiquitous sensors, making IoT widespread (Pramanik et al. 2019). The IoT architecture is organized into three fundamental layers conceptually. A. Application Layer, B. Transport or Network Layer, C. Sensing or Perception Layer (C).

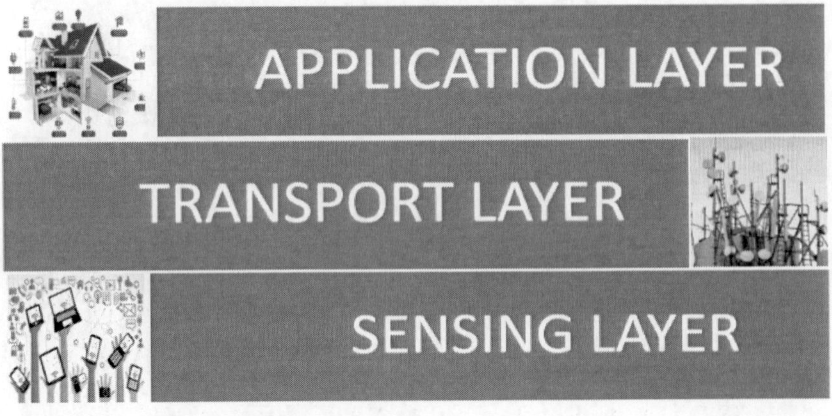

Figure 2. General Architecture of IoT.

2.1. Sensing Layer

In a layered fashion, the Sensing or Perception Layer is at the bottom of all the levels. Physical devices and components with built-in communication technology, such as smart gadgets, make up the sensing layer (Tervonen et al. 2010). (RFID, sensors, actuators, etc.). The perception layer's major goal is to link items to an IoT network and use deployed smart devices to measure, gather, and process sensed data before sending it to the upper layer via layer interfaces. To communicate with each other, these layers have standardized interfaces (Sethi and Sarangi 2017). This IoT architecture explains two types of interfaces: one between "Perception Layer" and "Transport Layer", and the other between "Transport Layer" and "Application Layer".

2.2. Transport Layer

The transport or network layer is a fundamental layer that is largely associated with the internet, as specified by the OSI reference model or the TCP/IP protocol suite (Alhamedi et al. 2015). The data transmission to and from the levels above and below it is handled by this layer. In IoT architecture, the Transport Layer serves as an intermediate layer. As with the TCP/IP network and the Internet (N. M. Kumar and Mallick 2018), this is also known as the network layer. The network, transport, and Internet layers are all interwoven in a three-layer design. This is why the Internet of Things uses a layered design, which allows layers to be added and combined easily. The transport layer receives the sensing layer's processed data and establishes the routes and channels for distributing it over integrated networks to the IoT hub, devices, and applications. Routing data packets is handled by the transport layer, which means routing protocols are implemented there. In IoT architecture, the network layer/transport layer is the most important layer since it combines several devices (Kwelwa 2018) ("hubs", "switches", "gateways", and so on) and communication protocols ("ZigBee", "Bluetooth", "Wi-Fi", "3G", "4G", "Long-Term Evolution" (LTE), and so on) (Garcia et al. 2018). The transport or network layer has two types of interfaces: one for connecting to lower layers and another for communicating with higher layers. All of the logic is built up to interact with a number of networks and devices that use a variety of communication technologies and protocols.

2.3. Application Layer

The Application Layer is the uppermost layer in an IoT layered architecture. Because it is where all of the logic is implemented, the business layer is another name for the application layer (Yassein, Shatnawi, and Al-Zoubi 2016). The application layer receives data from the transport layer and uses it to conduct the relevant services or activities. An application layer's function is to deliver services to the layers underneath it. Storage service for backing up data to a database, as well as an analysis service for analyzing received data and forecasting the condition of physical devices in the future (Mohamed 2019) are examples of these services. The application layer accepts data from the layers above it and makes services available to them (Nastase 2017). Only one interface is sandwiched with it in the application layer because it only communicates with the layer below it.

3. IoT Enabling Technologies and Protocols

Diverse suppliers have different technologies in the market due to the heterogeneity of IoT devices with different technologies. All of the enabling technologies must be integrated in order for devices to communicate with each other. The IoT is a wide-area network that uses industry-standard communication protocols (Al-Fuqaha 2013). Transducers (Sensor/Actuator) integrated with communication technology communicate via wired or wireless networks, typically utilizing the same Internet Protocol (IP) as the internet. The IoT is not always a component of the real internet (local).

3.1. Transducer

A device consisting of hardware and software that has the ability to transform one form of energy into another. Transducers come in a variety of shapes and sizes, depending on the application. There are two types of transducers in the IoT: sensor and actuator (SCME 2014). Sensor: a device that converts physical values to electrical output, or perceived data into an electrical signal. Sensors are the most common IoT devices with built-in communication capabilities. Actuator: a device that turns an electrical signal into a physical output (Rathod 2019). In other words, an actuator accepts input from a sensor (directly or indirectly) to make a physical change.

3.2. Radio Frequency Identification (RFID)

The IoT relies heavily on RFID tags. RFID tags are commonly used for identifying anything automatically & provide each thing or object a unique digital identity, allowing them to be deployed in networks and linked to digital data and services (Kosmatos, Tselikas, and Boucouvalas 2011). Active and passive RFID tags (Tan et al. 2018) are the two types of RFID tags. Because they communicate with the reader's interrogation signal, passive RFID tags do not require a battery. Passive tags are included in a range of items, including bank cards and road toll tags, which were among the first to be utilized globally. Active RFID readers include a built-in battery and are capable of communicating with tags like monitoring tags.

3.3. Wireless Sensor Networks (WSN)

WSN is a data-transmission-capable network communication medium. Wireless Sensor Networks and RFID devices can operate together to keep track of items. WSNs may be used in a variety of industries, including healthcare, government, and environmental services, and seismic sensing (Ghayvat et al. 2015). WSN could also be combined with RFID systems to connect physical and digital devices. They can accomplish objectives such as gathering information on their location, position, movement, temperature, and so forth. The most widely used WSN nowadays is based on the IEEE 802.15.4 standard (Dutta 2019), which is designed primarily for low-power sensors.

3.4. Addressing

The ability to detect Things in a unique way is critical for the IoT's success. The only method to identify and manage billions of devices remotely via the internet is to use addresses (Gubbi et al. 2013). Reliability, uniqueness, scalability, and persistence are the most crucial benefits of uniquely addressing. Every connected object, as well as those that have not yet been linked, must be individually identifiable in terms of position and functionality. IPv4 may not be able to support this huge number of items separately, but it may be able to identify a group as a single device (Kumar Gandhi and Kameswara Rao 2016). Due to the heterogeneity of "wireless nodes", different data formats, parallel operations, and data convergence from objects worsen the issue. The addressing protocol architecture of IPv6 (Savolainen, Soininen, and Silverajan 2013) gives more address space than a drop of water in the sea. According to some estimates, it may reach as high as 1030 addresses per individual. An IoT device may receive a worldwide IP address considerably more easily using IPv6, allowing for efficient peer-to-peer connectivity.

The IoT encompasses all forms of connections, such as "device to device", "device to person", and "person to person", implying massive connectivity of individuals (Gubbi, Buyya, and Marusic 2013). The current IoT trend can also allow the interconnection of objects and objects in order to create smart surroundings. The ability to uniquely identify things is crucial for a successful Internet of Things outcome in this regard. This is because addressing the enormous number of objects in a unique way is essential for controlling them through the Internet. The above-mentioned uniqueness idea, as well as dependability, scalability, and persistence, are all necessary conditions for developing a unique addressing method.

3.5. Protocols

There are a variety of protocols available, some of which can be deployed to IoT devices, but others may not be appropriate for this circumstance. In information and communication technology, A protocol is a set of guidelines for communicating in general (Tournier et al. 2020). In the context of IoT, communication can take three forms:

- Device to Device (D2D or M2M) communication: In the IoT, devices can communicate with one another. For this, the "Data-Distribution Service for Real-Time Systems" (Yang et al. 2012) (DDS) protocol is employed.
- Device to Server (D2S): Because data created by IoT devices must be transferred to a server, a protocol that can perform a task is required. MQTT ("Message Queuing Telemetry Transport") (Soni and Makwana 2017) is a protocol that accepts data from a device and sends it to a server. XMPP ("Extensible Messaging and Presence Protocol") (Çorak et al. 2018) is another protocol for connecting gadgets and people. It's a unique instance of the D2S pattern.

Table 1. IoT elements and protocols

IoT Elements		Samples
Identification	**Naming**	“EPC”, “uCode”
	Addressing	“IPv4”, “IPv6”
Sensing		“Smart Sensors”, “Wearables”, “Sensing devices”, “Embedded Devices”, “Sensors”, “Actuators”, “RFID tags”
Communication		“RFID”, “NFC”, “UWB”, “Bluetooth”, “BLE”, “IEEE 802.15.4”, “Z-Wave”, “Wi-Fi”, “WiFiDirect”, “LTE-A”
Computation	**Hardware**	“Smart Things”, “Arduino”, “Phidgets”, “Intel Galileo”, “Raspberry Pi”, “Gadgeteer”, “BeagleBone”, “Cubieboard”, “Smartphones”
	Software	OS (“Contiki”, “TinyOS”, “LiteOS”, “RiotOS”, “Andriod”) Cloud (“Nimbits”, “Hadoop”, etc.)
Service		“Identity-Related” (shipping), “Information Aggregation” (smart grid), “Collaborative-Aware” (smart home), “Ubiquitous” (smart city)
Semantic		“RDF”, “OWL”, “EXI”

Protocols		
Application Layer.		“DDS”, “CoAP”, “AMQP”, “MQTT”, “MQTT-SN”, “XMPP”, “HTTP”.
Service Discovery.		“mDNS”, “DNS-SD”
Infrastructure Protocols	**Routing Protocol.**	“RPL”
	Network Layer.	“6LoWPAN”, “IPv4/IPv6”
	Link Layer	“IEEE 802.15.4”
	Physical/ Device Layer	“LTE-A”, “EPCglobal”, “IEEE 802.15.4”, “Z-Wave”.
Influential Protocols		“IEEE 1888.3”, “IPSec”, “IEEE 1905.1”

- Server to Server (S2S): In an Internet of Things scenario, the server must also communicate device data with other servers. The "Advanced Message Queuing Protocol" (AMQP) (Naik 2017) is a server-to-server protocol that establishes the standard for middle-layer communication.

3.6. Summary of Findings

After examining a large amount of literature on the topic of the Internet of Things, numerous researchers have worked on architectures, applications, Communication Technology, and Protocols. We created a table that outlines the most important features and protocols defined by these organizations. Samples and protocols for IoT elements are separated into four distinct categories: "application", "service discovery", "infrastructure", and other "influential protocols". Table 1: IoT Elements and Protocols, provides a high-level overview of IoT architecture elements.

4. Applications Areas of IoT

The Potential of IoT makes it possible to think about developing a massive number of applications. From an enormous set of applications, only a little part is currently available to our public. There are many application domains and environments in which new IoT-based applications would likely improve and ease the way of our lives. For instance, at home, while traveling, in the health sector, workplace, transport sector, etc. The following papers have discussed most of the application areas of IoT (Al-Fuqaha et al. 2015)(Sethi and Sarangi 2017)(Singh and Singh Tomar 2019)(Hassija et al. 2019). These can be grouped but are not limited to the following domains as represented in Figure 3: Application Areas of IoT.

4.1. Smart City

There is no commonly agreed meaning of the term "smart city". The aim and goal are to make better use of public resources while cutting operating costs and improving the quality of services provided to the general public. It is characterized as a city that examines and integrates the status of all of its major facilities, such as "roads", "bridges", "tunnels", "rail/subways", and "airports", in order to better utilize its resources while providing the best possible service to its residents (Mohapatra and Panda 2019). A communication infrastructure that gives unique and simple access to a variety of public services, enhancing transparency for citizens, can help an urban IoT deployment fulfill the smart city's core goal (Arasteh et al. 2016). Indeed, the optimization of conventional public services such as transportation and parking, lighting, monitoring and maintenance of public places, cultural heritage preservation, trash collection, and hospital and school well-being might all benefit from an urban IoT (Zanella et al. 2014). Many national governments have announced plans to use ICT to manage public affairs, bringing the so-called Smart City concept to life. In June 2015, India announced a programme to upgrade urban centres fundamental infrastructure, which was started by Prime Minister Narendra Modi (Mir and Ravindran 2017). Each city will receive 1,000 crores in central government money to enhance its infrastructure under this programme.

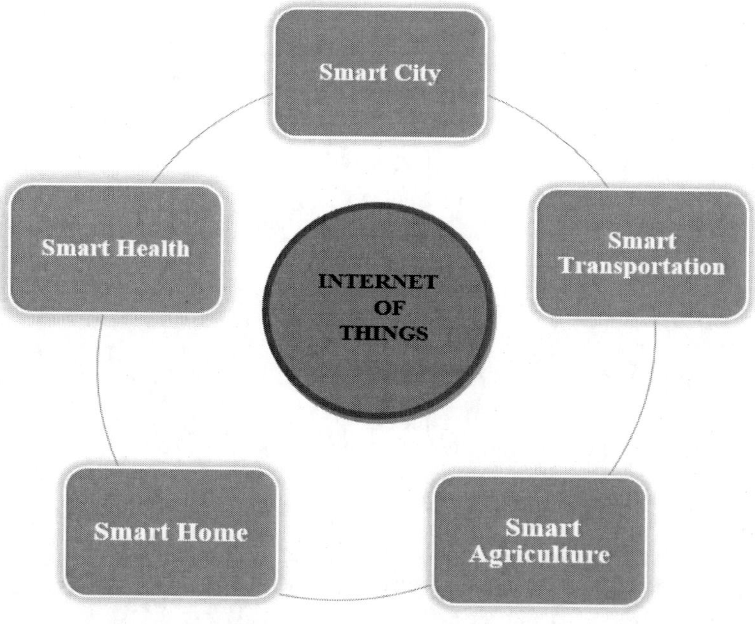

Figure 3. Applications of IoT.

4.2. Smart Transportation

Internet of things (IoT) is transforming every field, and smart transportation is one of them. It is a network of connected vehicles, roadways, etc. (Saarika P S, Sandhya K 2017) through a wireless network. Intelligent transportation will reshape and automate the roadways, railways, and airways. Smart transportation will also optimize cargo services and will create new business opportunities (Redhat 2016). By implementing IoT in vehicles, more excellent safety, reliability can be achieved. Smart parking, vehicle tracking are other applications of the intelligent transportation system (Muthuramalingam et al. 2019).

4.3. Smart Agriculture

Most of the population depends on agriculture directly or indirectly. Due to the population explosion, agricultural land is decreasing day by day. It is hard to feed the whole population using traditional ways of agriculture (Gondchawar and Kawitkar 2016). The new ways should be adopted so that production can be increased to provide food to the people. IoT is a promising technology that can be integrated with agriculture to make it smart. Smart agriculture uses the latest information communication tools to increase agricultural products' quality and quantity (Salim and Mitton 2020). Various sensors are available like temperature, humidity, moisture, light, water, etc. which can collect data and share it using WSN. Smart irrigation, smart farming, smart monitoring are sub-application domains of smart agriculture (Klerkx, Jakku, and Labarthe 2019).

4.4. Smart Home

As information and communication technology has progressed, many new sectors have evolved. One of these is the smart home, in which all electronic gadgets such as lighting, air conditioners, fans, and televisions may be controlled remotely via smartphones or laptops (Ahmadi et al. 2019). Smart gadgets are appliances that contain at least some form of connectivity technology and are installed in houses. Bluetooth, Wi-Fi, WiMax, 3G, 4G, LTE, and 5G are examples of radio access (RAN). (Tuli, Tuli, Tuli, et al. 2020) are primary building blocks for smart homes. In smart homes, sensors are deployed that sense the environment and share data with applications to respond accordingly (Li et al. 2021). In smart homes, even doors and windows are opened using actuators. "Smart energy", "smart surveillance" and "smart lighting" are sub-application areas of smart homes.

4.5. Smart Health

The IoT provides feasible solutions to many applications like traffic congestion, waste management, health, and emergency services. IoT has redesigned the traditional healthcare system by deploying smart objects and devices everywhere (Ahmadi et al. 2019). Electronic health record (EHR) is readily available due to the introduction of technology. Remotely health monitor, Adult care, fitness programs are attractive application areas of smart health. IoT-based healthcare systems are projected to save costs while also improving and enriching the user experience. There are a lot of medical devices and sensors available in the market (Tuli, Tuli, Wander, et al. 2020). Temperature, BP, HR, Oxygen saturation sensor, etc. are some medical sensors used in patient monitoring. Many applications are available like google fit, health assistant, cardiax, etc. available on smartphones (Li et al. 2021).

5. Challenges and Issues

The IoT is a network of "physical objects", "vehicles", "buildings", and other items with embedded "hardware", "software", "sensors", "actuators", and "network connectivity" that collect and share data (Gartner, n.d.). It is also one of today's fastest-growing technologies, promising a lot in terms of bringing the virtual world together and making it a waking reality. As a result, IoT devices may assist organizations in collecting and analysing large volumes of data, allowing them to make better and faster decisions, giving them a competitive advantage.

However, it has some limitations as it presents security challenges in identity management and usability concerns. Other important limitations include privacy concerns, widespread cyber threats, and unsolicited intrusions. Of note, privacy concerns are the most concerning issues. The information that is transferred becomes open access to the data collectors, government agencies, and hackers. Quite often, personal information gets passed on to non-intended persons and might be misused and finally causing security breaches. Moreover, challenges and issues in IoT are discussed in (Hassanalieragh et al. 2015) (Yaqoob et al. 2017) (Patel and Keyur 2016) (Lin et al. 2017) (Singh and Singh Tomar 2019).

6. Smart Healthcare System

A Smart Healthcare System is a network of Medical IoT (MIoT) devices, wearables, and sensors that are connected by any communication method. Patients' data is collected via a smart healthcare system, which is then analyzed to produce results (Javaid and Khan 2021). One of the most appealing application areas for the internet of things is medical and healthcare. Many medical applications, such as remote health monitoring, cardiovascular disorders, and geriatric care, can benefit from the Internet of Things (Rath and Pattanayak 2019). Wearable gadgets, such as smart wristwatches, heart rate monitors, pulse rate monitors, and BAN devices, are commonly employed to continually monitor patients (Rahman and Hossain 2021). The IoT healthcare system has a vast number of application areas, including the following but not limited to:

6.1. IoT Based Digital Telehealth

The "Internet of Health Things" (IoHT) is a subset of the IoT that attempts to link humans to medical facilities via communication technologies in order to monitor patients' vital signs. Telemedicine is becoming increasingly popular in rural areas that have limited access to healthcare services (Tsiouris et al. 2020).

6.2. IoT Based Ambulance

Using IoT-assisted ambulances, remote medical professionals recommend necessary measures to the medical team dealing with the patient, which is a viable alternative. This results in prompt patient reaction and successful patient management (Khan and Alam, n.d.).

7. Current Approaches and Future Scope

The "Internet of Things Security Foundation" (IoTSF) was founded on September 23, 2015, at the Digital Catapult in London to address growing security problems (IoTSF, n.d.). To overcome this harmful issue, network guards and firewalls have been utilized as network security devices, and they have been found to solve the problem to a higher extent. The base device platform analysis, network traffic verification, functional security requirements verification, and end-to-end penetration test are among the others. However, no comprehensive answer has been proposed thus far, necessitating the development of competent remedies to privacy concerns. Targeting data encryption, network traffic data, and end-to-end penetration testing would be an innovative strategy to putting an end to most privacy issues. The articles (Alieyan et al. 2019)(Internet of Robotic Things: Current Technologies, Applications 2021), (S. A. Kumar, Vealey, and Srivastava 2016) elaborate on the majority of potential directions. Any area can benefit from IoT, which can be combined with machine learning, deep learning, and artificial intelligence to deliver greater insights (Khanday et al. 2020).

Conclusion

This survey paper seeks to provide a thorough overview of IoT, including enabling technologies, architecture, and applications. A recent literature study was conducted in this chapter to examine all aspects of the Internet of Things that have been covered thus far, including architectures, supporting technologies, features and applications, concerns and obstacles, and future prospects. The fast expansion of smart devices necessitates the development of future IoT network architecture. Existing network topologies are unable to support the present number of smart devices, which is likely to grow in the future years. Existing protocols are bulky and consume a lot of resources, necessitating the adoption of new security mechanisms. This study discussed IoT application areas and their potential. IoT is still in its infancy, and much study needs to be done in this subject before it can be completely developed. In addition, this study discussed the IoT's future reach and open research issues. Because of its wide range of applications and heterogeneous mix of various communications and embedded technology in its architecture, the IoT has created a plethora of new opportunities for researchers, industrialists, and researchers in embedded, computer science, and information technology.

References

Ahmadi, Hossein, Goli Arji, Leila Shahmoradi, Reza Safdari, Mehrbakhsh Nilashi, and Mojtaba Alizadeh. 2019. *The Application of Internet of Things in Healthcare: A Systematic Literature Review and Classification. Universal Access in the Information Society.*, Vol. 18. Springer Berlin Heidelberg. https://doi.org/10.1007/s10209-018-0618-4.

Al-Fuqaha, Ala. 2013. "AL-FA-Internet of Things: A Survey on Enabling Technologies, Protocols, and Applications." *IEEE Communication Surveys & Tutorials (Accepted for Publication)*, 1 (2): 78–95. https://doi.org/10.5752/P.2316-9451.2013v1n2p78.

Al-Fuqaha, Ala, Mohsen Guizani, Mehdi Mohammadi, Mohammed Aledhari, and Moussa Ayyash. 2015. "Internet of Things: A Survey on Enabling Technologies, Protocols, and Applications." *IEEE Communications Surveys and Tutorials*, 17 (4): 2347–76. https://doi.org/10.1109/COMST.2015.2444095.

Alhamedi, Adel H., Hamoud M. Aldosari, Václav Snášel, and Ajith Abraham. 2015. "Internet of Things Communication Reference Model and Traffic Engineer System (TES)." *Advances in Intelligent Systems and Computing*, 334: 303–13. https://doi.org/10.1007/978-3-319-13572-4_25.

Alieyan, Kamal, Ammar Almomani, Rosni Abdullah, Badr Almutairi, and Mohammad Alauthman. 2019. "*Botnet and Internet of Things (IoTs)*," no. January: 304–16. https://doi.org/10.4018/978-1-5225-9742-1.ch013.

Arasteh, H., V. Hosseinnezhad, V. Loia, A. Tommasetti, O. Troisi, M. Shafie-Khah, and P. Siano. 2016. "Iot-Based Smart Cities: A Survey." *EEEIC 2016 - International Conference on Environment and Electrical Engineering*, no. May. https://doi.org/10.1109/EEEIC.2016.7555867.

Atzori, Luigi, Antonio Iera, and Giacomo Morabito. 2010. "The Internet of Things: A Survey." *Computer Networks*, 54 (15): 2787–2805. https://doi.org/10.1016/j.comnet.2010.05.010.

Bhuvaneswari, V., and R. Porkodi. 2014. "The Internet of Things (IOT) Applications and Communication Enabling Technology Standards: An Overview." *Proceedings - 2014 International Conference on Intelligent Computing Applications, ICICA 2014*, no. March: 324–29. https://doi.org/10.1109/ICICA.2014.73.

CERP-IOT. 2008. "Internet of Things Strategic Research Roadmap - European Commission." *Aerospace Technologies and Applications for Dual Use*, no. January: 9. http://ec.europa.eu/information_society/policy/rfid/documents/in_cerp.pdf.

Çorak, Burak H., Feyza Y. Okay, Metehan Güzel, Şahin Murt, and Suat Ozdemir. 2018. "Comparative Analysis of IoT Communication Protocols." *2018 International Symposium on Networks, Computers and Communications, ISNCC 2018*, no. June. https://doi.org/10.1109/ISNCC.2018.8530963.

Dutta, Dushyanta. 2019. *IEEE 802.15.4 as the MAC Protocol for Internet of Things (IoT) Applications for Achieving QoS and Energy Efficiency. Lecture Notes in Networks and Systems.*, Vol. 31. Springer Singapore. https://doi.org/10.1007/978-981-10-8911-4_14.

Garcia, Laura, Jose Miguel Jiménez, Miran Taha, and Jaime Lloret. 2018. "Wireless Technologies for IoT in Smart Cities." *Network Protocols and Algorithms*, 10 (1): 23. https://doi.org/10.5296/npa.v10i1.12798.

Gartner. n.d. "Gartner Internet Of Things (Iot)." Https://Www.Gartner.Com/En/Information-Technology/Glossary/Internet-of-Things.

Ghayvat, Hemant, Subhas Mukhopadhyay, Xiang Gui, and Nagender Suryadevara. 2015. "WSN- and IOT-Based Smart Homes and Their Extension to Smart Buildings." *Sensors* (Switzerland), 15 (5): 10350–79. https://doi.org/10.3390/s150510350.

Gondchawar, Nikesh, and R. S. Kawitkar. 2016. "IoT Based Smart Agriculture." *International Journal of Advanced Research in Computer and Communication Engineering*, 5 (6): 838–42. https://doi.org/10.17148/IJARCCE.2016.56188.

Gubbi, Jayavardhana, Rajkumar Buyya, and Slaven Marusic. 2013. "1207.0203." *Atmospheric Environment*, no. 1: 1–19. https://doi.org/10.1016/j.future.2013.01.010.

Gubbi, Jayavardhana, Rajkumar Buyya, Slaven Marusic, and Marimuthu Palaniswami. 2013. "Internet of Things (IoT): A Vision, Architectural Elements, and Future Directions." *Future Generation Computer Systems*, 29 (7): 1645–60. https://doi.org/10.1016/j.future.2013.01.010.

Hassanalieragh, Moeen, Alex Page, Tolga Soyata, Gaurav Sharma, Mehmet Aktas, Gonzalo Mateos, Burak Kantarci, and Silvana Andreescu. 2015. "Health Monitoring and Management Using Internet-of-Things (IoT) Sensing with Cloud-Based Processing: Opportunities and Challenges." *Proceedings - 2015 IEEE International Conference on Services Computing, SCC* 2015, 285–92. https://doi.org/10.1109/SCC.2015.47.

Hassija, Vikas, Vinay Chamola, Vikas Saxena, Divyansh Jain, Pranav Goyal, and Biplab Sikdar. 2019. "A Survey on IoT Security: Application Areas, Security Threats, and Solution Architectures." *IEEE Access*, 7: 82721–43. https://doi.org/10.1109/ACCESS.2019.2924045.

Internet of Robotic Things: Current Technologies, Applications, Challenges and Future Directions. 2021. "Internet of Robotic Things: Current Technologies, Applications, Challenges and Future Directions." http://arxiv.org/abs/2101.06256.

"IoT End User Perceptions, Strategies and Preferences in Hungary." 2018, no. April.

IoTSF. n.d. "Internet of Things Security Foundation Set for Global Launch." Https://Www.Iotsecurityfoundation.Org/Donec-at-Mauris-Enim-Duis-Nisi-Tellus/#:~:Text=The%20Internet%20of%20Things%20Security,Security%20excellence%20in%20IoT%20systems.

Islam, S. M.Riazul, Daehan Kwak, Md Humaun Kabir, Mahmud Hossain, and Kyung Sup Kwak. 2015. "The Internet of Things for Health Care: A Comprehensive Survey." *IEEE Access*, 3: 678–708. https://doi.org/10.1109/ACCESS.2015.2437951.

Ivanov, Andre. 2014. "The Internet of Things." *IEEE Design and Test*, 31 (3): 4–5. https://doi.org/10.1109/MDAT.2014.2335314.

Javaid, Mohd, and Ibrahim Haleem Khan. 2021. "Internet of Things (IoT) Enabled Healthcare Helps to Take the Challenges of COVID-19 Pandemic." *Journal of Oral Biology and Craniofacial Research*, 11 (2): 209–14. https://doi.org/10.1016/j.jobcr.2021.01.015.

Khan, Samiya, and Mansaf Alam. n.d. "*IoT Based Traffic Management System for Ambulances*," 0–5.

Khanday, Akib Mohi Ud Din, Syed Tanzeel Rabani, Qamar Rayees Khan, Nusrat Rouf, and Masarat Mohi Ud Din. 2020. "Machine Learning Based Approaches for Detecting COVID-19 Using Clinical Text Data." *International Journal of Information Technology (Singapore)*, 12 (3): 731–39. https://doi.org/10.1007/s41870-020-00495-9.

Klerkx, Laurens, Emma Jakku, and Pierre Labarthe. 2019. "A Review of Social Science on Digital Agriculture, Smart Farming and Agriculture 4.0: New Contributions and a Future Research Agenda." *NJAS - Wageningen Journal of Life Sciences*, 90–91 (November): 100315. https://doi.org/10.1016/j.njas.2019.100315.

Kosmatos, Evangelos A., Nikolaos D. Tselikas, and Anthony C. Boucouvalas. 2011. "Integrating RFIDs and Smart Objects into a UnifiedInternet of Things Architecture." *Advances in Internet of Things*, 01 (01): 5–12. https://doi.org/10.4236/ait.2011.11002.

Kumar Gandhi, Baratam M., and M. Kameswara Rao. 2016. "A Prototype for IoT Based Car Parking Management System for Smart Cities." *Indian Journal of Science and Technology*, 9 (17). https://doi.org/10.17485/ijst/2016/v9i17/92973.

Kumar, Nallapaneni Manoj, and Pradeep Kumar Mallick. 2018. "The Internet of Things: Insights into the Building Blocks, Component Interactions, and Architecture Layers." *Procedia Computer Science*, 132: 109–17. https://doi.org/10.1016/j.procs.2018.05.170.

Kumar, Sathish Alampalayam, Tyler Vealey, and Harshit Srivastava. 2016. "Security in Internet of Things: Challenges, Solutions and Future Directions." *Proceedings of the Annual Hawaii International Conference on System Sciences*, 2016-March: 5772–81. https://doi.org/10.1109/HICSS.2016.714.

Kwelwa, S D. 2018. "Please Note : Changes Made as a Result of Publishing Processes Such as Copy-Editing, Formatting and Page," 1–5.

Ladd, Ted, and Olaf Groth. 2015. "The Internet of Things." *Economist (United Kingdom)*, 411 (8964).

Li, Wei, Yuanbo Chai, Fazlullah Khan, Syed Rooh Ullah Jan, Sahil Verma, Varun G. Menon, Kavita, and Xingwang Li. 2021. "A Comprehensive Survey on Machine Learning-Based Big Data Analytics for IoT-Enabled Smart Healthcare System." *Mobile Networks and Applications*. https://doi.org/10.1007/s11036-020-01700-6.

Lin, Jie, Wei Yu, Nan Zhang, Xinyu Yang, Hanlin Zhang, and Wei Zhao. 2017. "A Survey on Internet of Things: Architecture, Enabling Technologies, Security and Privacy, and Applications." *IEEE Internet of Things Journal*, 4 (5): 1125–42. https://doi.org/10.1109/JIOT.2017.2683200.

Madakam, Somayya, R. Ramaswamy, and Siddharth Tripathi. 2015. "Internet of Things (IoT): A Literature Review." *Journal of Computer and Communications*, 03 (05): 164–73. https://doi.org/10.4236/jcc.2015.35021.

Mir, Mahmood Hussain, and D. Ravindran. 2017. "Role of IoT in Smart City Applications : A Review." *International Journal of Advanced Research in Computer Engineering Technology*, 6 (7): 1099–1104.

Mohamed, Khaled Salah. 2019. "The Era of Internet of Things." *The Era of Internet of Things*, 93–111. https://doi.org/10.1007/978-3-030-18133-8.

Mohapatra, Badri Narayan, and Prangya Prava Panda. 2019. "Machine Learning Applications to Smart City." *ACCENTS Transactions on Image Processing and Computer Vision*, 5 (14): 1–6. https://doi.org/10.19101/tipcv.2018.412004.

Muthuramalingam, S., A. Bharathi, S. Rakesh kumar, N. Gayathri, R. Sathiyaraj, and B. Balamurugan. 2019. "Iot Based Intelligent Transportation System (Iot-Its) for Global Perspective: A Case Study." *Intelligent Systems Reference Library*, 154: 279–300. https://doi.org/10.1007/978-3-030-04203-5_13.

Naik, Nitin. 2017. "Choice of Effective Messaging Protocols for IoT Systems: MQTT, CoAP, AMQP and HTTPNaik, N. (2017). Choice of Effective Messaging Protocols for IoT Systems: MQTT, CoAP, AMQP and HTTP. In 2017 IEEE International Symposium on Systems Engineering, ISSE 2017 -." *2017 IEEE International Symposium on Systems Engineering, ISSE 2017 - Proceedings*, 1–7. http://ieeexplore.ieee.org/document/8088251/.

Nastase, Lavinia. 2017. "Security in the Internet of Things: A Survey on Application Layer Protocols." *Proceedings - 2017 21st International Conference on Control Systems and Computer, CSCS 2017*, no. July 2016: 659–66. https://doi.org/10.1109/CSCS.2017.101.

Of, Internet, and Smart Cities. 2018. "ITU-T."

Patel, K, and Keyur. 2016. "Internet of Things-IOT: Definition, Characteristics, Architecture, Enabling Technologies, Application & Future Challenges." *Universidad Iberoamericana Ciudad de México*, no. May.

Pfeifer, Tom. 2012. "The Internet of Things - A White Paper," no. July. http://www.tom-pfeifer.name/academic/publish/Internet_of_Things_White_paper_Pfeifer.pdf.

Pramanik, Pijush Kanti Dutta, Bijoy Kumar Upadhyaya, Saurabh Pal, and Tanmoy Pal. 2019. *Internet of Things, Smart Sensors, and Pervasive Systems: Enabling Connected and Pervasive Healthcare. Healthcare Data Analytics and Management*. Elsevier Inc. https://doi.org/10.1016/b978-0-12-815368-0.00001-4.

Rahman, Md Abdur, and M. Shamim Hossain. 2021. "An Internet of Medical Things-Enabled Edge Computing Framework for Tackling COVID-19." *IEEE Internet of Things Journal*. https://doi.org/10.1109/JIOT.2021.3051080.

Rath, Mamata, and Binod Pattanayak. 2019. "Technological Improvement in Modern Health Care Applications Using Internet of Things (IoT) and Proposal of Novel Health Care Approach." *International Journal of Human Rights in Healthcare*, 12 (2): 148–62. https://doi.org/10.1108/IJHRH-01-2018-0007.

Rathod, Vivek T. 2019. "A Review of Electric Impedance Matching Techniques for Piezoelectric Sensors, Actuators and Transducers." *Electronics (Switzerland)*, 8 (2). https://doi.org/10.3390/electronics8020169.

Ray, P. P. 2018. "A Survey on Internet of Things Architectures." *Journal of King Saud University - Computer and Information Sciences*, 30 (3): 291–319. https://doi.org/10.1016/j.jksuci.2016.10.003.

Redhat. 2016. "Intelligent Systems for the Transportation Industry." *Technology Overview*, 1–7. https://www.redhat.com/cms/managed-files/iot-transportation-technology-overview-201608-en.pdf.

Saarika P S, Sandhya K, Sudha T. 2017. "6Pduw 7Udqvsruwdwlrq 6\Vwhp Xvlqj,R7." 978-1-5386-0569-1$31.00 c?2017 IEEE 6: 1104–7.

Salim, Christian, and Nathalie Mitton. 2020. "Machine Learning Based Data Reduction in WSN for Smart Agriculture." *Advances in Intelligent Systems and Computing*, 1151 AISC: 127–38. https://doi.org/10.1007/978-3-030-44041-1_12.

Savolainen, Teemu, Jonne Soininen, and Bilhanan Silverajan. 2013. "IPv6 Addressing Strategies for IoT." *IEEE Sensors Journal*, 13 (10): 3511–19. https://doi.org/10.1109/JSEN.2013.2259691.

SCME. 2014. "Introduction to Transducers, Sensors, and Actuators." *Southwest Center for Microsystems Education (SCME) University of New Mexico*, 4. http://engtech.weebly.com/uploads/5/1/0/6/5106995/more_on_transducers_sensors_actuators.pdf.

Sethi, Pallavi, and Smruti R. Sarangi. 2017. "Internet of Things: Architectures, Protocols, and Applications." *Journal of Electrical and Computer Engineering*, 2017. https://doi.org/10.1155/2017/9324035.

Singh, Kaptan, and Dr Deepak Singh Tomar. 2019. "Architecture, Enabling Technologies, Security and Privacy, and Applications of Internet of Things: A Survey." *Proceedings of the International Conference on I-SMAC (IoT in Social, Mobile, Analytics and Cloud), I-SMAC 2018*, 642–46. https://doi.org/10.1109/I-SMAC.2018.8653708.

Soni, Dipa, and Ashwin Makwana. 2017. "A Survey on Mqtt: A Protocol of Internet of Things(IoT)." *International Conference on Telecommunication, Power Analysis and Computing Techniques (Ictpact - 2017)*, no. April: 0–5. https://www.researchgate.net/publication/316018571_A_SURVEY_ON_MQTT_A_PROTOCOL_OF_INTERNET_OF_THINGSIOT.

Tan, Ping, Han Wu, Peng Li, and He Xu. 2018. "Teaching Management System with Applications of RFID and IoT Technology." *Education Sciences*, 8 (1). https://doi.org/10.3390/educsci8010026.

Tervonen, Jouni, Mika Luimula, Sakari Pieskä, Tomi Pitkäaho, and Juha Alaspää. 2010. "RFID and Wireless Sensor and Actuator Networks in Advanced Production Applications." *Solid State Phenomena*, 164 (June): 155–60. https://doi.org/10.4028/www.scientific.net/SSP.164.155.

Tournier, Jonathan, François Lesueur, Frédéric Le Mouël, Laurent Guyon, and Hicham Ben-Hassine. 2020. "A Survey of IoT Protocols and Their Security Issues through the Lens of a Generic IoT Stack." *Internet of Things*, 100264. https://doi.org/10.1016/j.iot.2020.100264.

Tsiouris, Kostas M., Dimitrios Gatsios, Vassilios Tsakanikas, Athanasios A. Pardalis, Ioannis Kouris, Thelma Androutsou, Marilena Tarousi, et al. 2020. "Designing Interoperable Telehealth Platforms: Bridging IoT Devices with Cloud Infrastructures." *Enterprise Information Systems*, 14 (8): 1194–1218. https://doi.org/10.1080/17517575.2020.1759146.

Tuli, Shreshth, Shikhar Tuli, Rakesh Tuli, and Sukhpal Singh. 2020. "Since January 2020 Elsevier Has Created a COVID-19 Resource Centre with Free Information in English and Mandarin on the Novel Coronavirus COVID- 19 . The COVID-19 Resource Centre Is Hosted on Elsevier Connect, the Company's Public News and Information," no. January.

Tuli, Shreshth, Shikhar Tuli, Gurleen Wander, Praneet Wander, Sukhpal Singh Gill, Schahram Dustdar, Rizos Sakellariou, and Omer Rana. 2020. "Next Generation Technologies for Smart Healthcare: Challenges, Vision, Model, Trends and Future Directions." *Internet Technology Letters*, 3 (2): e145. https://doi.org/10.1002/itl2.145.

Vermesan, O., Friess, P., Guillemin, P., Gusmeroli, S., et al. n.d. "Internet of Things Strategic Research Agenda." *Internet of Things—Global Technological and Societal Trends*.

Yang, Jinsong, Kristian Sandstrom, Thomas Nolte, and Moris Behnam. 2012. "Data Distribution Service for Industrial Automation." *IEEE International Conference on Emerging Technologies and Factory Automation, ETFA*. https://doi.org/10.1109/ETFA.2012.6489544.

Yaqoob, Ibrar, Ejaz Ahmed, Ibrahim Abaker Targio Hashem, Abdelmuttlib Ibrahim Abdalla Ahmed, Abdullah Gani, Muhammad Imran, and Mohsen Guizani. 2017. "Internet of Things Architecture: Recent Advances, Taxonomy, Requirements, and Open Challenges." *IEEE Wireless Communications*, 24 (3): 10–16. https://doi.org/10.1109/MWC.2017.1600421.

Yassein, Muneer Bani, Mohammed Q. Shatnawi, and Dua' Al-Zoubi. 2016. "Application Layer Protocols for the Internet of Things: A Survey." *Proceedings - 2016 International Conference on Engineering and MIS, ICEMIS 2016*, no. September: 1–4. https://doi.org/10.1109/ICEMIS.2016.7745303.

Zanella, Andrea, Nicola Bui, Angelo Castellani, Lorenzo Vangelista, and Michele Zorzi. 2014. "Internet of Things for Smart Cities." *IEEE Internet of Things Journal*, 1 (1): 22–32. https://doi.org/10.1109/JIOT.2014.2306328.

Chapter 3

Towards the Smart Diagnosis of Brain Disorders Using Artificial Intelligence

Waseem Ahmad Mir[1], Izharuddin[1], Tawseef Ayoub Shaikh[2] and Junaid Ali Reshi[1]

[1]Department of Computer Engineering, Aligarh Muslim University, Aligarh, India

[2]Department of Computer Engineering, Pandit Deendayal Energy University, Gujrat, India

Abstract

Brain, the most vital part of the human body comprising of the cerebrum, cerebellum, and brainstem. The human brain is the central organ of the nervous system; it controls and manages the activities of the body while coordinating with other parts of the body by processing and integrating information from sensory organs. It is the decision-making unit of the human body. There are many disorders associated with the brain which are either genetic or are caused due to age by the death of brain cells. The most common brain disorders are Alzheimer's disease, Parkinson's disease, Epilepsy, Down syndrome, stress, migraine, dementia, etc. To understand the inner activities of the brain, and to diagnose the malfunctions of the brain, some non-invasive techniques have been made available. One of the most common techniques to understand activities of the brain is to measure the electrical activity of the brain. This is done by using Electroencephalogram (EEG). Similarly, many imaging techniques are being used to understand the structure of the brain which includes MRIs, PET scans, etc. With the advance in technology and modern ICT, big volumes of data in the form of brain signals and images are available in hospitals and online data houses. The secondary use of

In: AI-Enabled IoT for Smart Health Care Systems
Editors: Tawseef Ayoub Shaikh, Tabasum Rasool and Mohammed Wasid
ISBN: 978-1-68507-977-2

this data has revealed promising results in the diagnosis of brain abnormalities using Artificial Intelligence. An ample number of techniques in the machine learning domain have been developed to retrieve meaningful information. In the future, it is hoped that these developments in ICT will help medical professionals in the diagnosis of brain-related disorders and the development of Brain-Computer Interfaces with accurate models. This chapter will explain in detail the underlying technologies and will deliberate upon some of the machine learning techniques which have shown promising results in classification tasks.

Keywords: brain disorders, machine learning, deep learning, LSTM, RNN, neurology

1. Introduction

Brain, the most vital organ of the human body is basically, a nerve tissue. Brain is the coordination center of the body which integrates sensory information, regulates various systems of the body, and directs information flow in the form of motor responses. In general brain is the learning and coordination center of the body. The brain is composed of billions of neuron cells. Electrical and chemical messages generated in the neuron cells are transmitted from one neuron to another neuron through junctions known as synapses. These electrical and chemical transmissions, basic to sensory functions play an essential role in memory management, thinking capability, and learning process. Abnormal functioning of the brain leads to various types of neural disorders. These disorders affect the normal working of the human body thus limiting their daily activities and restricting their participation in the normal functioning of society. Brain disorders affect the central and peripheral nervous systems. Some of the common disorders include Epilepsy, Parkinson's disease (PD), Alzheimer’s disease (AD), dementia, migraine, multiple sclerosis, neuro-infections, brain tumors, traumatic disorders, etc. The normal and abnormal activities of the brain can be measured using many techniques which include signal analysis using Encephalogram recordings, image analysis using MRI recordings, and many pathological tests. EEG is one of the most commonly used diagnostic techniques in brain disorder detection and diagnosis. An enormous amount of data is available in the form of EEG signals and MRIs in health institutions. The secondary use of this data will hopefully yield many promising results if this data is analyzed in a modern way using newer technologies. One of these newer technologies is Artificial Intelligence, a recent computer-aided technique that has revolutionized many social sectors including healthcare. It is hoped that Artificial Intelligence techniques at the back of which are Machine learning (ML) and Deep Learning (DL) algorithms will produce results very accurate in the prediction and diagnosis of many health ailments including neural disorders. Before going into the details of AI and its use in making healthcare smart, let us briefly discuss some of the common brain disorders and the traditional methods of diagnosing them.

2. Brain Disorders

Brain disorders in general are brain-related disorders affecting the central and peripheral nervous system. At the global level, hundreds of millions of people suffer from brain-related disorders. Brain disorders pose a very chronic health challenge at the global level. One of the reasons for this massive challenge is that services related to neurological disorders are massively disproportionate to the severity of the problem. It is believed that in times coming forth healthcare providers may witness an unprecedented rise in brain disorders, especially in underdeveloped and developing countries. A study conducted by World Health Organization concludes that the impact of brain-related disorders on society has been underestimated [1]. The high rate of morbidity and mortality among the patients suffering from brain disorders speaks volumes about the need for effective diagnostic approaches and subsequent treatment. An effective means to overcome this problem is to integrate clinical data with modern AI systems to discover disease subtypes and categorize them according to the severity of the disease. Diagnosis in neural disorders has remained limited to symptoms and observable signs observed by the clinicians. With recent advances in artificial intelligence, new insights in the neurosciences categorize normal and abnormal functioning of the brain in a, more precise and accurate way. The convergence of brain sciences with AI technology is expected to revolutionize precision medicine thus addressing the constraints in both research and practice. The learning processes in AI systems continuously rewire themselves into new learning functions which are imperative to understand the various aspects of the brain dysfunctions associated with the neural disorders. Before going into the details of applications of AI in healthcare, especially in understanding and diagnosis of brain disorders, let us first discuss some commonly occurring brain disorders in brief.

2.1. Epilepsy

Epilepsy is described by the occurrence of unprovoked Epileptic seizures one of the most common brain disorders. Epilepsy in a literal sense can be expressed solely by recurrent seizures. Epileptic seizures occur as a result of a plethora of acute metabolic imbalances and severe brain insults. It is very difficult to make a distinction between provoked and unprovoked seizures in low-profile medical settings. Epilepsy is not age-specific; it can occur at all ages. In children, the number of epileptic cases has fallen over the last few decades in developed countries [2]. It is estimated that over 50 million people are currently suffering from epilepsy worldwide and 7.7 million people are being added to this number annually. Owing to this huge number the diagnosis of Epilepsy remains vital to the clinicians. Neurophysiological and brain imaging investigations are being used to diagnose the syndrome. The brain images in the form of MRIs coupled with diagnosis using AI is producing promising results in identifying the structural and functional causes of the disease.

2.2. Alzheimer's Disease

Alzheimer's disease which figures highest among all brain disorders is usually the most common precursor of dementia [3]. It has assaulted mankind at a very rapid pace. It is characterized by the manifestations of loss of memory and cognitive dysfunctions. Globally 15 million people are suffering from Alzheimer's disease. The main precursors of Alzheimer's disease are cortical amyloid plaques and neurofibrillary tangles. Alzheimer's is found in all countries, races, and cultures. In developing countries like India, for example, AD in most of cases is not considered as a medical anomaly rather it is seen as part of normal aging in adults. The common symptoms are aggression, sleep disturbances, wandering, anxiety, depression, hallucinations, and delusions. AI advances may provide better solutions for the diagnosis of AD. They may provide accurate and less error-prone results as part of a reliable diagnostic system and possibly help in the early detection of the disease. AI systems generally use structural images of the brain based on MRI scans for diagnosis and detection of AD.

2.3. Parkinson Disease

Parkinson's Disease (PD), the second most prevalent brain disorder affects 2-3% of the adult population above 60 years of age, affecting their quality of life. It is caused due to the progressive degradation of neural tissue in the substantia nigra part of the nervous system which in turn causes striatal dopamine deficiency [4]. The common symptoms include difficulty in speaking, writing, and gait abnormalities. For detection of PD speech, gait and EEG analysis are carried out, however, speech analysis is the most common way of investigating diagnosis. Several techniques have been developed to diagnose PD at the earliest stage, however recent advances in AI and expert systems in healthcare have developed various software tools based on machine learning algorithms for accurate diagnosis and detection of the disease. These techniques are non-invasive and help in telemonitoring, predictive analysis, thus ameliorating the quality of life of the patients.

2.4. Multiple Sclerosis

Multiple Sclerosis is chronic, a most common autoimmune nontraumatic neurological disorder affecting the nervous system. It attacks the myelinated axons in the central nervous system. Around 3.5 million people in the US are suffering from Multiple Sclerosis and half of them have problems in walking. It is unpredictable and highly varied among the patients. Most of the patients suffer episodes of reversible brain deficits, followed by neuron deterioration over time. The number of patients suffering from Multiple Sclerosis is increasing globally impacting the socio-economic setup of the countries. Since complex gene-environment plays a significant role in the spread of this disease, but the causes and mechanisms behind the rapid increase in the disease remain a mystery. The induction of precision medicine and predictive analysis using machine learning algorithms is expected to yield good results in the diagnosis of the disease.

2.5. Migraine

Migraine is the most common yet unknown headache. It is a perplexing brain disorder in which brain tissues play an implicit role during the attack. Sometimes it is a debilitating disorder representing an interaction between inputs from the peripheral and central nervous system and trigeminovascular system and the cerebral cortex. The most common symptoms of migraine are frequent urination, sensitivity to light and sound, nausea, vomiting, aura, blurry vision, throbbing pain, and lack of sleep. Migraine dominates 60% of the women and 30% of men wasting about 70 lack hours due to the severity of pain. In recent times many ML techniques have been developed for the automatic prediction and classification of migraine

3. Artificial Intelligence

Artificial Intelligence (AI), one of the advanced branches of Computer Science (CS) attempts to understand and develop intelligent software programs which can learn based on experience and help to predict a calculated outcome. AI has gradually changed the landscape of many social sectors, healthcare being one of them. Healthcare and biomedical research especially neuroscience with the use of AI has emerged into prominence at the scientific level as breakthroughs at the diagnostic level are happening at a breakneck pace. AI technologies in collaboration with technological giants like Google have started clinical practice with medical institutions. One such example is the University of Iowa recognized by the US Food and Drug Administration (FDA) developing a model for diagnosing severe to moderate Diabetic retinopathy (DR). The term Artificial Intelligence traces back to 1956 when it was used the first time. Although significant progress in the development of AI was made in the last few decades but it was only after 2012 when a successful resurgence of AI, led to the development of important image classifiers [5]. Post this, AI is a well-recognized research area and its success is reaching new heights making it impossible to track the progress it is making. In the healthcare industry the success of AI from the last few decades of the last century put forth some important breakthroughs with the introduction of auto interpretation of electrocardiograms, electroencephalograms, etc. Considered as the back burners of AI in medicine and healthcare, AI in healthcare is expected to make promising breakthroughs in the fields of disease diagnosis, prediction medicine, and the making of biomarkers.

Researchers have proposed systems and developed them into clinical decision support systems emphasizing the interpretation of clinical reasoning, disease diagnosis, and appropriate treatments. In recent times AI has found applications in medical diagnostic systems in both image and signal analysis which was previously done by medical experts. It is hoped that this continues to make progress in other healthcare facilities like translational health research and clinical practice [6]. Previously disease diagnosis and medication relied on the medical expertise of the healthcare professionals which used to be based on robust decision rules simplistically. AI in healthcare has leveraged learning algorithms that can look at complex interactions, identifying correlated data, and identify patterns from the data. Based on these formulations the task of classification and subsequent decision making is automated with precision far better than the health experts. A typical AI system used for disease diagnosis is shown in Figure 1.

Some of the basic terms in Artificial Intelligence and their explanation are given below.

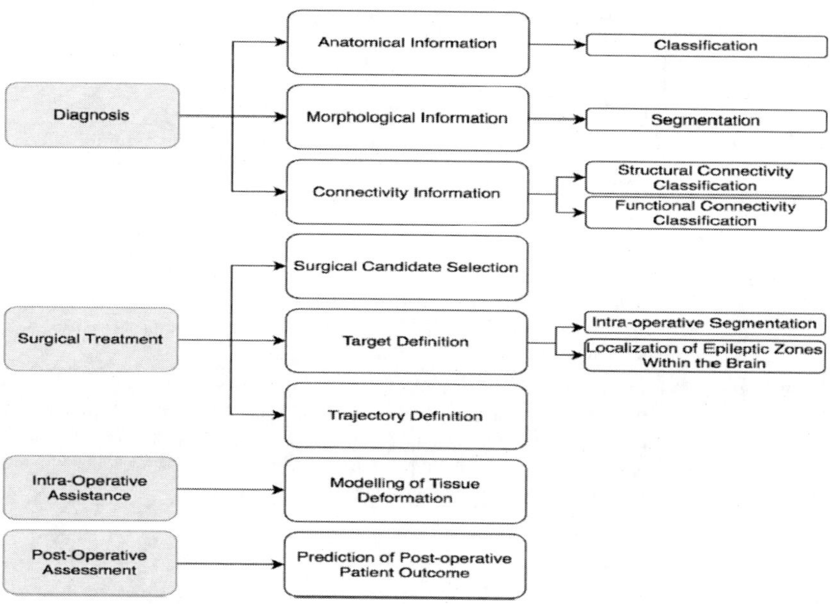

Figure 1. An example of an AI system

Table 1. Important terms in AI and their explanation

Artificial Intelligence	The term Artificial Intelligence means the use of computers to devise intelligent models with minimum human intervention. It is the branch of Computer science used for analytics of big data and to extract meaningful information from the data.
Machine Learning (ML)	Machine Learning (ML) is the subset of Artificial Intelligence (AI) that addresses the question of developing systems that improve automatically through learning. The learning algorithms are supervised unsupervised, semi-supervised, and active learning. Machine learning, a growing field in technology relies on the intersection of computer science and statistics.
Supervised Learning	Supervised ML, a subset of machine learning, constructs algorithms capable of producing general patterns by feeding externally supplied data to predict the fate of unseen data. These are classification algorithms for the categorization of data from prior knowledge. Some examples are Decision trees (DTs), Bayesian networks, K-nearest neighbor (KNN), Support vector machines (SVM), etc.
Unsupervised Learning	Unsupervised learning, also known as clustering is based on ML algorithms that are capable of analyzing unlabelled data. These algorithms find hidden groupings in the unlabelled data, ideal for customer segmentation and image recognition. Some examples are hierarchal clustering, k-means clustering, probabilistic clustering, etc.
Reinforcement Learning	Reinforcement learning trains a machine to make a decision sequence to reach a conclusion in an uncertain and complex environment. The machine employs trial and error method to come up with a solution in an intelligent way by reward and penalty method,
Artificial Neural Network	The term Artificial Neural Networks (ANNs) or simply Neural Networks (NNs) mean Machine learning (ML) algorithms modeled based on the functionality of the biological brain and realized on a structure made of input, hidden, and output layers
Deep Learning	Deep Learning (DL) is a special class of machine learning (ML) based on representation-based learning. The name deep actually reflects the bulk of hidden layers in the Artificial Neural Network (ANNs). The network learns and extracts inherent most relevant features from successive hidden layers.
Precision Medicine	Precision medicine is a promising and targeted approach for effective treatment. Contrary to traditional assessment of a complex health condition precision medicine relies on health data for decision making and subsequent treatment paths to be followed. It provides a basis for planning large studies improving disease diagnosis.

4. Healthcare and AI

In recent times there is a lot of hype about Artificial Intelligence and its applications in healthcare. AI has introduced artificially intelligent technologies in healthcare. The technology is being used to automate routine tasks, assist in hospital care and improve clinical research and digitize the healthcare system. In the present COVID era AI has paved many ways to develop new models, thereby exploring new avenues for medicines, developing vaccines, and improving healthcare outcomes. It is believed that AI can augment human performance whilst improving efficiency, accuracy, and productivity for both healthcare professionals and patients. The applications of AI in healthcare are wide and will eventually cover diagnostics and operational technologies. Clinical applications of AI have demonstrated improved efficiency in image and signal analysis which is expected to save billions of dollars in the future. Although the use of AI in clinical diagnosis is still in the infancy stage but results emerging from some reputed research institutes indicate that AI-based diagnosis is at par with the performance of tested experts, demonstrating the competence level of AI models. Table 2 shows some of the applications of AI in healthcare.

Table 2. Applications of AI in healthcare

Robot-Assisted Surgery	AI-based Robot-Assisted surgeries help speed up surgeries while making delicate incisions without fatigue in crucial procedures. New surgical models can be built by using data from past surgeries reducing the accidental and unintended movements during the surgeries.
Diagnosis	AI-assisted diagnostic systems are modeled to diagnose diseases precisely and with faster speed. It is expected to help doctors to detect diseases more accurately and make the diagnosis more cost effective.
Healthcare Administration	AI is playing a healthcare administration role by managing medical data, records, billing, consultation, and many more services pivotal to hospital management.
Automated Image diagnosis	AI employed models have been used to transform complex visual observations in the form of medical images into machine learning techniques that can help in exploring new insights from the data and coming up with advanced clinical practices.
Clinical Participation	AI is capable of transforming the key steps of clinical trials towards the improvement of trial success rates which lowers the cost of research and design.
Nursing Assistants	AI-based Nursing Assistants offer personalized care to the patients. They identify diseases based on symptoms, the health status of patients and eventually schedule appointments with the concerned doctors.
Clinical Decision Support System	Using Natural Language Processing, health professionals can extract the relevant and useful information from the medical records of the patients, thus helping them in their clinical decision system.

4.1. Artificial Intelligence for Brain Disorders

Artificial Intelligence has specifically in the brain domain achieved promising results in the diagnosis of disorders, prediction, postoperative assessment, and planning by making use of AI techniques like Artificial Neural Networks (ANNs) and classical machine learning (ML) algorithms like support vector machines, random forest. These approaches have risen to prominence among the widely used analytical tools because of their capability to solve specific problems. The most common types of data used in AI-based analysis are brain images and signals. Since the predictions are solely dependent on data fed to the system, it is therefore very important to collect the most comprehensive data for quantitative and qualitative characterization studies. One of the most important benefits of using AI in brain disorder diagnosis is that the procedure paves a way for disease prediction in a fast and non-invasive manner. Advances in signal and image processing technologies have further made the analysis cost effective. The manual interpretation of brain signals and images is time consuming and susceptible to human errors. The error rate and misjudgments only in radiology are greater than 3-5%, therefore AI-based novel methods and techniques help physicians and health professionals in effectively analyzing the data. Furthermore, the computational power of the AI systems has increased tremendously with the inclusion of GPUs, therefore advanced use of AI algorithms on complex and voluminous data has increased, producing significant results. Machine Learning Algorithms (ML) which are a subset of AI algorithms perform best while automatically "learning" to classify conditions of the brain that address brain problems. ML techniques comprise of many steps ranging from data pre-processing, feature extraction, feature selection, ranking, dimensionality reduction, and classification. These Algorithms are being used to detect the brain disorders like seizures, epilepsy, Alzheimer's disease, Multiple Sclerosis (MS), and degenerative diseases. Before discussing some ML algorithms used in brain disorder diagnosis, let us have a brief look at the data types used in AI-based Brain Disorder diagnosis.

4.2. Types of Data

To understand the working and structure of the brain in a non-invasive manner, images of the brain in the form of MRIs and signals in the form of EEG are being deployed. Innovations in these techniques have improved the field of diagnostics and prediction medicine. Table 3 explains in brief various types of brain images and signals.

Table 3. Types of Biomedical Data for Brain Disorder Diagnosis

Brain Images	
MRI (magnetic resonance imaging)	Magnetic resonance (MRI) is a noninvasive imaging technique that uses a strong magnetic field and radio waves to create detailed images of the organs and tissues within the body.
PET (positron emission tomography)	Positron emission tomography (PET) scan reveals the biochemical and metabolic functions of tissues and organs using an imaging test. Radioactive drug tracers identify the normal and abnormal functioning of the organs.
CT (computed tomography)	Computed tomography is a computerized x-ray imaging technique used to get detailed images (cross sectional images and slices) of the body noninvasively for disease diagnosis.
IUS (intra-operative ultrasound)	The intraoperative ultrasound technique works on high energy sound waves to generate sonograms (images) of the body that can help the surgeons to find the normal and abnormal functioning of the body.
fNIRS (functional near-infrared spectroscopy)	Functional near infrared spectroscopy (fNIRS) is a diagnostic technique that can detect the change of hemoglobin inside the organ by finding differences in optical absorption. It is noninvasive in nature.
HSI (Hyper-spectral imaging)	Hyper-spectral imaging (HSI) is also an imaging modality, based on the collection of electromagnetic spectral information over 2 dimensional and three-dimensional space having applications diagnosis and automated surgery.
Brain Signals	
EEG (electroencephalography)	Electroencephalography (EEG) is usually non-invasive method used for measuring, recording, and interpreting the electrical activities of the brain. If the signals are recorded from intracranial parts, then invasive techniques are used to record the activities of the brain.
MER (Microelectrode Recording)	Microelectrode Recording (MER) is a diagnostic technique used for recording electrical patterns and structures from surrounding brain structures.

5. ML Algorithms for Brain Disorder Diagnosis

In this section, we will discuss some of the basic Machine Learning (ML) algorithms that are being used for the detection and diagnosis of brain disorders.

5.1. Support Vector Machines (SVMs)

Support Vector Machine (SVM), a supervised machine learning algorithm that learns by example and assigns labels to the objects is one of the most commonly used techniques in Machine Learning. SVMs require labeled data for the classification of unknown data. The decisions are made based on hyperplanes and decision boundaries. A hyperplane separates the data points into different categories. SVM is a mathematical entity and it maximizes a mathematical function with respect to some given data points i.e., input data. To understand the working of an SVM machine we need to understand the basic four aspects of SVM

1. Separating hyperplane or Decision boundary: It separates the set of data points into different classes.
2. Maximum margin hyperplane: It means the hyperplane that has the maximum distance between the hyperplane and the training observations.
3. Soft Margin: Since the data points are not always linearly separable and may contain errors. To overcome this limitation a soft margin parameter is introduced which specifies a tradeoff between hyperplane errors and the size of the margin.
4. Kernel function: When data is not linearly separable and no single point can separate two classes, the kernel function adds an additional dimension, so that data becomes separable resulting in high dimensional space.

SVMs are very powerful learning models which can be applied for both regression and classification. It can handle both continuous and categorical data. For the classification purpose, the objective function maps the training data to 'higher dimensional space' introducing a 'linear hyper plane' after identifying a maximum margin. Figure 2 illustrates an SVM in which an optimal hyperplane separates a group of instances.

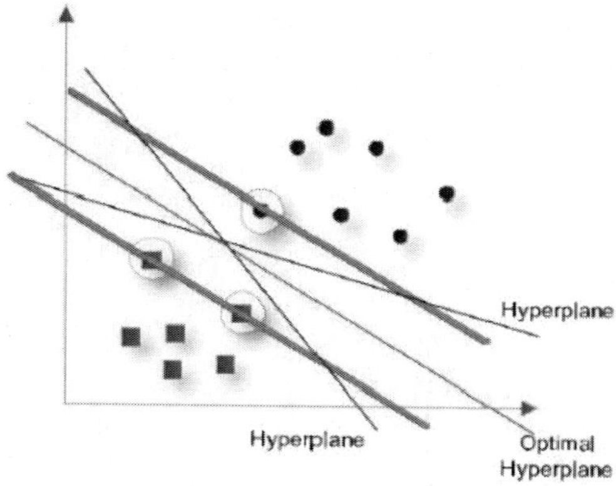

Figure 2. Example of SVM.

5.2. K-Nearest Neighbor (K-NN)

K-Nearest Neighbour(K-NN) is a supervised learning non-parametric ML algorithm applied for both classification and regression problems. K-NN keeps all training examples in memory and when unseen instance *x* is fed, it looks from *k* similar examples already fed to the system and returns with the majority label in case of classification and an average label in case of regression problems. It is instance-based learning i.e., event related, a part of lazy learners which labels the instances based on the previously known similar problems. In k-NN architecture, no computation is done before the query is given to the system. The similarity of the two examples is given by a distance function. Classification of groups can be done using different distance metrics like Euclidean distance, Manhattan distance (MhD), and Minkowski distance (MnD). Hamming distance is more frequently used for labeling the instances which are continuous in nature. Whenever an unseen data point is fed to the learning system, it classifies it by voting the neighbors, which means the data point is grouped among k- nearest neighbors measured by the distance function given by different distance metrics

$$Euclidean = \sqrt{\sum_{i=1}^{k}(x_i - y_i)^2}$$

$$Manhattan = \sum_{i=1}^{k} |x_i - y_i|$$

$$Minkowski = \left(\sum_{i=1}^{k} (|x_i - y_i|)^q \right)^{1/q}$$

6. Deep Learning Algorithms for Brain Disorder Diagnosis

The last decade has witnessed the use of deep learning in a wide range of applications. Deep learning, which is a subset of Artificial Intelligence (AI) is based on Artificial Neural Networks (ANNs) having excellent model building capability, for problems valid over a wide range of areas. DL algorithms have become very popular in recent years for image classification, object detection, text classification. In the medical field, it can be used in neurology, pathology, pulmonology, muscular and abdominal studies Training in deep learning networks is done with more than two non-output layers [7]. Deep Learning networks comprise of an input layer, a finite set of hidden layers and finally, an output layer of processing units called output neurons [8]. The two biggest challenges in Machine learning namely exploding gradient and vanishing gradient have to some great extent got solved using backpropagation. Backpropagation is an efficient algorithm that uses hyperbolic tangent for computing gradients in networks using the chain rule.

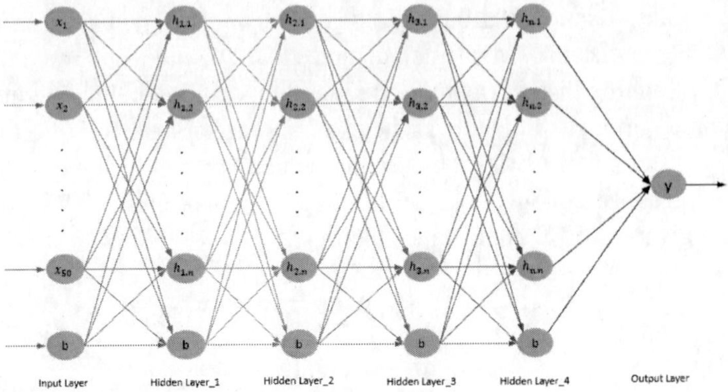

Figure 3. DNN architecture.

An input layer is followed by a deep dense layer. The dense layer also known as the hidden layer consists of neurons, where most of the processing takes place. It defines the learning behavior of the model. Following the dense layer or the hidden layer, we have an output layer that consists of output nodes depending on the number of predefined classes of the data. Pertinently this number is problem specific. For two classes, "binary classification", there is only one output node that corresponds to the predicted class. Similarly, "multiclass classification" requires n no of output nodes for n predicted classes. Here *n* represents the no of labeled classes in the data. There are no specific rules to determine the number of layers in the hidden layer. The task at hand usually determines the no. of hidden layers. There is internal communication between the neurons in the hidden layer. We usually apply nonlinearity on the input neurons, then the output produced is the mathematical manipulation of the input data. Firstly we assign weights to the input neurons which keep on updating during the learning phase. We calculate each output layer, which is then passed to the next input layer. Shallow networks i.e., the networks having less dense hidden layers are easy to train as compared to the deep networks which are computationally powerful and have a wide range of applications in natural language processing, image (NLP) and speech recognition, computer vision, etc. Figure 3 shows the architecture of Deep Neural Network.

6.1. Convolutional Neural Networks

Convolutional Neural networks (CNN) are commonly used deep neural networks that significantly reduce the number of parameters without losing the quality of the model in terms of its performance metrics. The name convolution is derived from mathematical linear operation convolution (of two matrixes). CNNs were built with image processing in mind, they have several layers which include a convolutional layer (parametric), non-linearity layer (non-parametric), pooling layer (non-parametric), fully connected layer (parametric), and the output layer. The performance of CNN is excellent because they enable learning which is data driven, representative, and trains on remarkably sufficient training data. However, obtaining large datasets in medical imaging remains a challenge. Some of the most common applications of CNN are in computer vision, natural language processing, image, and signal processing [9]. Besides transfer learning, there are mainly three techniques involved in the employment of CNNs to image processing and consequent classification. First, training the Convolutional Neural Network (CNN) from scratch, second, using CNN on pre trained features, and third, unsupervised CNN with supervised fine tuning.

6.1.1. Working of CNN

Convolutional neural networks (CNNs) are fed with input, where initial processing takes pace, then it is fed to the dense hidden layer, where feature extraction takes place and finally output layer classifies it under different categories. An image as input to the CNN sees it as an array of pixels depending on the resolution of the image. CNN recognizes it as

$$h*w*d$$

((h = Height, w = Width, d = Dimension). The input passes through a series of convolutional layers with filters (Kernels), pooling, and fully connected layers (FC). After the convolution, a SoftMax function at the output layer is used to classify an object with values ranging from 0 to 1. This classification is based on probabilistic modeling. The two most common CNN architectures are (a) LeNet, introduced first by Yan LeCun for bit recognition comprising of 5 convolutional, layers and one fully connected layer, and (b) Alex Net which comprises of 5 convolutional layers and as many as 2 fully connected layers. Max pooling layers are introduced at the first, second, and fifth convolutional layer. First, of this kind, this CNN proved that deep learning is effective in computer vision tasks. Some basic terms related to CNNs are discussed below.

(a) Convolution: Convolution is a mathematical operation that changes a function to something else. Convolution intertwines two types of information. It extracts the relevant features from the input data. It preserves the relationship between different pixels with the help of two inputs, an image matrix, and a filter, by learning features using small squares of input. In the process of convolution pixels in their respective fields are converted into a single value. The output of the convolutional layer is a vector. Convolutions have been used in image processing with different filters that can perform the tasks of edge detection, emboss, blur and sharpen by enforcing connectivity patterns between neurons and adjacent layers.

(b) Stride: Stride is the step size or the number of pixel shifts of the moving window (input matrix). It is assumed that the succeeding layer has a lot of overlapping with the preceding layer. This overlapping can be manipulated by controlling the stride size. When the stride is 1 the filter slides to the right and bottom, moving the filter to 1 pixel at a time. Stride 2 means the shift of 2 pixels at a time and so on. The figure below shows the stride of step size 2.

(c) Padding: One of the drawbacks of the convolution step is that the filter does not fit perfectly to an input image, therefore there may be some loss of information at the borders of the image. To resolve this, we can drop that part of the image where the filter does not fit. This keeps the only valid part of the image and drops the other portion. This process is called valid padding. Another method is to pad the image with zeros. This method is known as zero padding. It is a simple and efficient method to resolve the problem. This type of padding also manages the output size by preventing the network output from shrinking in depth.

6.2. Recurrent Neural Networks: Recurrent Neural

Recurrent Neural Networks (RNN) is widely used on NLP tasks to classify and generate sequences capturing long term and local dependencies. A sequence represents a matrix where rows represent feature vectors. The order of the rows matters. A special variant of RNN is Long Short-Term Memory (LSTM), which has been an effective model in a wide range of applications like language modeling, handwriting recognition, and generation graves. Unlike CNN, the recurrent neural network is not feedforward, but it contains loops. Each unit k of recurrent layer l contains a real state $h_{l,}\ k$. In other words, this state can be viewed as the memory of the unit. Each k in layer l receives 2 inputs, vector from previous layer l-1 and vector state from this same layer l from the preceding time step. Hidden state puts in memory, the information about the sequence. The feature vectors from the input are read sequentially by the network in order of time steps.

Recurrent neural network converts also known as RNNs are a subset of Neural Networks that allow previous outputs to be used as inputs by converging independent activations into dependant activations by providing the same weights and biases to all the layers. By doing this there is a considerable reduction in the complexity of parameters. By memorizing previous outputs and feeding each output as input to the proceeding layer, the weights are shared across time. Three layers can be joined together with the same weights and biases making it a single recurrent layer. The mathematical expression for calculating the current state is given by.

$$K_t = f(k_t\text{-}1, X_t)$$

where,
k_t = current state
k_{t-1} = previous state
x_t = input state
Usually, ***tanh*** and ***softmax*** are used as activation functions, but both of them suffer from vanishing gradient problem. Mathematically activation function is given by

$$k_t = \tanh(W_{kk}k_{t-1} + W_{xk}X_t)$$

where,
w_{kk}= weight at the recurrent neuron
w_{xk} = weight at input neuron
The output is calculated as.

$$Y_t = W_{ky}k_t$$

Y_t = output
W_{ky} = weight at the output layer

In RNN, we feed a single time step of the input to the network. We calculate the current state as a function of the set of current input and previous step. Time steps can be taken according to the nature of the problem for joining the information from several previous steps. The final current state represents the output. We compare this predicted output with the labeled output. The difference between the two is the error generated. This error is then backpropagated to update the network with a different weight, thereby training the network. The most common RNNs used in practice are gated RNNs. Long Short-Term Memory (LSTM) and gated recurrent unit (GRU) belong to this group. However, there remains the gradient vanishing and exploding problems, besides training RNN is a very difficult task.

7. Performance Metrics for Evaluation

For all healthcare applications using ML or DL the evaluation of performance metrics is very important in order to evaluate the overall performance of the particular algorithm. For a disease diagnosis model performance metrics represent different conclusions. We may have a model performing better in terms of accuracy but may have very poor specificity. The benchmark measures used for measuring the overall performance of the system are Accuracy, Sensitivity, Specificity, precision, Area Under the Curve Receiver operating characteristics, etc. We summarize these performance metrics in the table below.

8. Challenges in AI Development in Healthcare

There are many challenges to the development of AI in healthcare that need to be addressed. Below are some of the challenges that are explained in detail:

Table 4. Performance Metrics for Model Evaluation

Accuracy	Accuracy is an elementary metric to test the reliability of any classification system. It is given by the number of accurate diagnoses to the number of actual diagnosis made. Mathematically Accuracy = τp + τN/τp + FP + τN + FN where τP and τN are true positive and true negative respectively
Precision	Precision measures how proximate measurements of the same item are to each other which means it is possible to be very precise but not so accurate. Precision is independent of accuracy.
Sensitivity	Sensitivity measures the number of actual positive labels (true positive) that got predicted as positive. It is also called recall. Mathematically Sensitivity= τP/ τP + FN In other words, patients suffering from a disease are correctly predicted.
Specificity	Specificity is the ability of a machine to correctly classify an individual as disease free. Mathematically Specificity = τN /τN + FP
AUCROC	Area Under the Curve Receiver Operating Characteristic AUROC is a performance evaluation method used to differentiate between classes. The curve visualizes how much the machine is capable of distinguishing the classes. It defines the ability of the model to distinguish between the binary choices under diverse discrimination threshold

8.1. Errors and Injuries

AI systems might at times give wrong results, in healthcare systems where the life of an individual is at stake, if a wrong prediction is made, the result can be life threatening. Imagine a wrong drug suggested by an AI system or an error in predicting cancer in an MRI. While an error by a health care professional may put a single man's life at threat, but a wrong prediction by a machine can be fatal to thousands of patients.

8.2. Data Availability

AI systems require huge reserves of data to train upon from multiple sources. The data is usually acquired from pharmacies, electronic health records, insurance claim records, etc. This data is usually fragmented, complicated, and incomprehensible. Therefore, there is always a risk of making errors.

Patients usually have the leverage to consult different healthcare providers and can switch to different insurance companies, therefore data is usually fragmented, which makes it complicated and less comprehensible, ultimately adding the risk of errors and cost factor.

8.3. Privacy Concerns

Healthcare data is sensitive and there are possibilities of privacy breaches. AI has the capability to predict sensitive and revealing sensitive and personal information about the patients even when the patient has not provided the information. There needs to be a balance between providing data to data scientists and subsequently protecting the sensitive data from any misuse. New approaches are required to streamline the development of AI and secure the confidentiality and sensitivity of data.

8.4. Bias and Inequality

Since AI systems learn through data, there is the possibility that they can absorb biases present in the data. Clinicians and health professionals have raised concerns over automating the health sector over this issue. The biases in the AI healthcare system stem from historically biased practices which lead to biased data sets, lack of oversight, and bias of practitioners in recognizing it. Therefore, the best anti-bias training needs to be given to healthcare professionals.

8.5. This Could Lead to Shifts in the Profession

Automation of the health industry with sophisticated AI systems will lead to shifts in the medical profession. For example, in the field of radiology, if the work is fully automated, it will lead to a fall in human knowledge, making professionals fail to detect errors in AI systems.

Conclusion

In this chapter, a general overview of AI in healthcare is given with special emphasis on brain disorders. AI in healthcare is expected to enable accurate diagnosis and fast service by gradually bringing efficient theoretical solutions to various brain related disorders. Due to the huge data available, currently, effective algorithms have helped us significantly in understanding the structure and functionality of the brain. Deep learning a subset of machine learning performs well with large datasets. There is a growing importance of publicly available datasets as the deep learning algorithms perform well in practical settings and a large amount of data with variations is being generated regularly at the health facilities.

References

Administration UFaD. Guidance for industry: electronic source data in clinical investigations. 2013 https://www.fda.gov/downloads/drugs/guidance/ucm328691.pdf (accessed 1 Jun 2017).

Albawi, Saad; Mohammed, Tareq Abed; Al-Zawi, Saad (2017). *[IEEE 2017 International Conference on Engineering and Technology (ICET) - Antalya, Turkey (2017.8.21-2017.8.23)] 2017 International Conference on Engineering and Technology (ICET) - Understanding of a convolutional neural network., (), 1–6.* doi:10.1109/ICEngTechnol.2017.8308186.

D Rizvi, I Nissar, S Masood, M Ahmed, F Ahmad, "*An LSTM based Deep Learning model for voice-based detection of Parkinson's disease*", IJAST, vol. 29, pp. 337-343, 2020.

I Nissar, D Rizvi, S Masood, and A Mir, "*Voice-based detection of Parkinson's disease through ensemble machine learning approach: A Performance Study*", Phat 19(19): e2, vol. 5, pp. 1-8, 2020

I Nissar, W A Mir, Izharuddin, T A Shaikh "*Machine Learning Approaches for Detection and Diagnosis of Parkinson's Disease- A Review*", vol. 1, pp. 898-905, ICACCS 2021.

Jiang F, et al. *Stroke and Vascular Neurology* 2017; 2: e000101. doi:10.1136/svn-2017-000101.

Khan, P., Kader, M.F., Islam, S.R., Rahman, A.B., Kamal, M.S., Toha, M.U. and Kwak, K.S., 2021. Machine Learning and Deep Learning Approaches for Brain Disease Diagnosis: Principles and Recent Advances. *IEEE Access*, *9*, pp.37622-37655.

McCarthy, J., 2007. What is artificial intelligence?

Murray CJL, Lopez AD, eds. *The global burden of disease: a comprehensive assessment of mortality and disability from diseases, injuries and risk factors in 1990 and projected to 2020*. Cambridge, MA

Sander, Josemir W. The epidemiology of epilepsy revisited, Current Opinion in Neurology: April 2003 - Volume 16 - Issue 2 - p 165-170

Segato, A., Marzullo, A., Calimeri, F. and De Momi, E., 2020. Artificial intelligence for brain diseases: A systematic review. *APL Bioengineering*, *4*(4), p.041503.

Shaikh, Tawseef Ayoub, Rashid Ali, and Waseem Ahmad Mir. "An Intelligent Healthcare System for Automated Alzheimer's Disease Prediction and Personalized Care." *International Journal of Next-Generation Computing* 12.2 (2021

W.A. Mir, Izharuddin and I. Nissar, "Contribution of application of deep learning approaches on biomedical data in the diagnosis of neurological disorders: A review on recent findings," pp. 87-97, ICCISIoT, CCIS, 13-14 Dec 2019, Agartala India, springer, 2020.

Y. Bengio, "Practical recommendations for gradient-based training of Deep Architectures. Neural Networks: Tricks of the Trade," 2nd Edition, pp.437–478,2012.

Chapter 4

Machine Learning Techniques for IoT-Enabled Health Care Environment

Ayushi Chahal*, Preeti Gulia and Nasib Singh Gill
Department of Computer Science & Applications, Maharshi Dayanand University, Rohtak, Haryana, India

Abstract

Internet of Things (IoT) came out to be a robust platform that helps in connecting every domain of everyday life. Healthcare is one of the domains of the world which go hand in hand with state-of-the-art technologies. IoT has made a drastic change in the healthcare domain. Machine Learning plays a vital role in making healthcare system smart and automated environments. This paper attempts to address all the aspects of the healthcare domain, which may be significantly improved by exploiting IoT and machine learning. The paper presents the pros and cons of embedding IoT in the healthcare domain. The bibliometric analysis uses Scopus and Web of Sciences datasets for IoT-enabled Healthcare applications using Machine Learning techniques. As a result, most cited papers are collected, leading to targeted and specific studies. This study also covers different organizations of the world which have given their valuable time for research in this area. This study helps to analyze different Machine Learning algorithms used for healthcare applications like surgery, patient monitoring, disease prediction, etc. A 'heart failure prediction' dataset is used to study Machine Learning algorithms in an IoT healthcare environment. The dataset is firstly pre-processed by eliminating duplicates from it and balancing the imbalanced data. Accuracy, Recall, F1 score, and Precision are the metrics used for

*Corresponding Author's Email: ayushi.rs.dcsa@mdurohtak.ac.in.

In: AI-Enabled IoT for Smart Health Care Systems
Editors: Tawseef Ayoub Shaikh, Tabasum Rasool and Mohammed Wasid
ISBN: 978-1-68507-977-2

a comparative analysis of machine learning algorithms used in this study. Random Forest machine learning algorithm outperform the comparative algorithms.

Keywords: IoT, healthcare, machine learning, predictive analysis, IoMT

1. Introduction

Today, the Internet of Things (IoT) is the basic necessity that helps to connect various devices over different geographical locations. IoT sensor devices collect a massive amount of data that must get converted into valuable insights. Nowadays, the Internet of Things (IoT) has become a vast network of physical devices connected to one another through the internet. This network helps physical devices to communicate and transfer data with one another (A.K. Majumdar, 2019). Because of the expansion in implanted IoT gadgets in various physical devices, IoT has become progressively broad (K. Singh et al., 2017). The IoT gadgets use a few sensor gadgets that are ready to gather an enormous volume of information in various areas which is handled by AI methods to settle on the choice with regards to the help issues (H. Fouad et al., 2020). IoT sensor gadgets are viably used in various applications (P. Sethi et al., 2017), like healthcare frameworks, covering gadgets, clean home upkeep, indoor regulators, lighting installations, home apparatuses, and security frameworks. Domains of real-life which are highly affected by IoT technologies are shown in Figure 1.

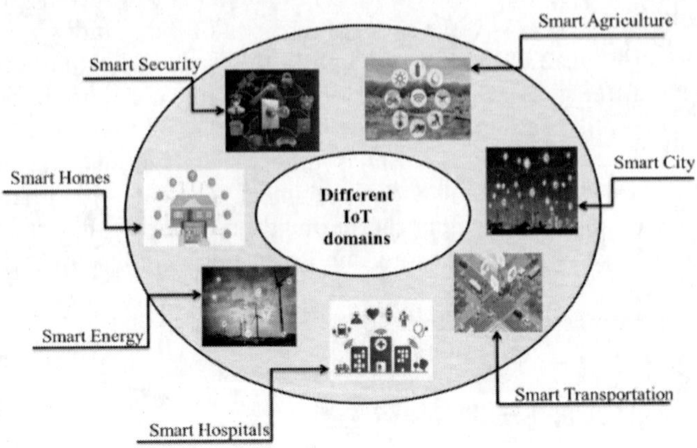

Figure 1. Different IoT Domains.

The Healthcare industry is a fast-growing and a very sensitive domain. IoT sensors are assumed as an essential part of the healthcare system in various applications (R. Pantelopoulos et al., 2010), that has countless medical care administrations. These progressions help the medical services to provide optimum care to their patients. The execution of IoT sensors in the medical care area improved the shared expectation among patients and specialist organizations. Additionally, this execution upgraded the therapy approaches. Also, the IoT sensor-based infection conclusion measure improved the nature of treatment adequately (F. Aktas et al., 2018).

Data about health care may originate from a variety of places, including the electronic health record (which contains lab findings, imaging tests, and diagnostic codes), activity trackers, and genetic testing, to name a few. Generally, healthcare data is real time Big data that is needed to be handled with care. ML is a statistical approach used for a learning process that helps in decision making or prediction. Deep learning models, a type of machine learning approach, have recently emerged as an example of a high-level approach. Since clinical information has become digitized, ML is assumed to be a significant part of the analysis of healthcare data. Analysts have investigated various machine learning models for prediction in the field of medical care framework in the previous decade (Farshad Firouzi et al., 2018).

2. Literature Review

Aidan Fuller et al. (2020) introduced readers to the new terminology "Digital Twin" which is a burning concept in various industries these days. Digital Twin is basically a balance and communication between physical and virtual machines. IoT and machine learning play a very important role in establishing this relationship in the Digital Twin scenario. Gayatri Gopal et al. (2019) have discussed the evolution of healthcare system from digital era to the intelligent era. Authors discussed how healthcare systems are upgrading themselves from time to time. Also, key components that are necessary for the applicability of intelligence into the healthcare systems are explained in detail, as shown in Figure 2.

Imran Khan et al. (2019) presented their work on Intelligent Healthcare Monitoring System (HMS). Authors used different sensors to measure blood pressure, body temperature, heart beat and ECG. Pi-camera and Aurdino UNO help in continuous monitoring of these sensor' data in the Raspberry-pi wifi network. Arduino UNO send sensor data collected through different IoT sensors to Raspberry-pi, which further sends data over the cloud database using the internet. This cloud data is being monitored by doctors and nurses on other end.

Ji-Peng Olivia Li et al. (2021) discussed IoT, ML and 5G tele-communication technologies that can be used for eye care problem detection challenges. The authors explained the role of Tele-health and artificial intelligence play in ophthalmologists' life. Authors have discussed new technologies that different nations are adopting to handle diabetic retinopathy, retinopathy of rashness, age-related macular degeneration, glaucoma, refractive mistake amendment, waterfall and other front fragment issues.

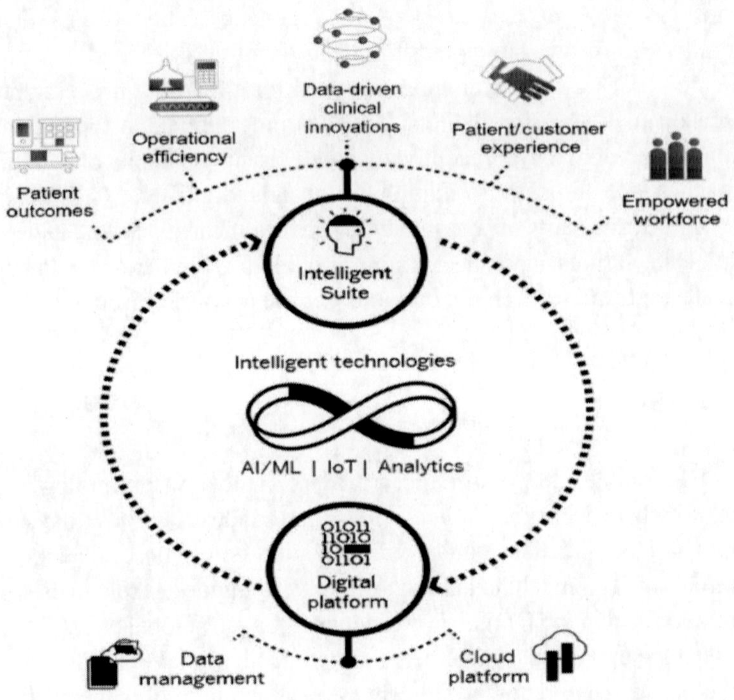

Figure 2. Smart Healthcare Framework [source: GayatriGopal et al. (2019)].

Yazdan Ahmad Qadri et al. (2020) presented to use a Network which is designed by software to improve the efficiency of the Healthcare Internet of Things (H-IoT). Internet of Nano Things (IoNT) and Tactile Internet (TI) topics are also discussed in the paper. It help to understand, how these technologies are helping H-IoT to boom at large scale. Xiaofeng Jin et al. (2020) discussed the challenges and prospects of using biosensors in IoT enabled healthcare environment. Authors have discussed the integration of wearable biosensors devices (like smart contact lenses, smart watches, saliva sensors, ring and sweat sensors, etc.) with artificial intelligence techniques like machine learning and deep learning.

Taisir Hasan Abdulameer et al. (2020) designed an IoT healthcare monitoring system to help elderly people. Charmi Jobanputra et al. (2019) also presented a survey on the health care monitoring system. In this study, authors have given an overview on the importance of machine learning models like decision trees, K-nearest neighbors, support vector machines, hidden Markov model and other deep learning models like artificial neural networks (ANNs), convolutional neural networks (CNNs) and recurrent neural networks (RNNs) for a health care monitoring system. The authors have discussed different sensor devices that can be used to gather datasets and have also presented some of the datasets that can be used for data analysis by the researchers. Hoa Hong Nguyen et al. (2017) presented a survey of healthcare monitoring applications for chronic disease for aged people. The authors presented a detailed study of converting IoT device data into clinical feedback. This methodology considers scope of viewpoints, including detecting, sending, preparing, putting away, mining and learning. This methodology assists in creating valuable and compelling insights from the data collected through improved frameworks of IoT medical services applications. The consequence of the survey tracked down that the development of IoT applications for medical services is in space of self-care, machine learning and mining the data.

Rahul Krishnan Pathinarupothi et al. (2019) presented a smart edge Healthcare system that is used to monitor remote patients with the help of small wearable sensors. These sensors transmit data on the cloud through the internet. This study declares that IoT is very fruitful in monitoring patients remotely to provide a hint and detect heart problems.

The utilization of IoT for ceaseless observation of general wellbeing is, as a rule, being embraced by different nations while creating a gigantic volume of heterogeneous, multisource, dynamic, and high-speed information. Dealing with a particularly tremendous measure of high-velocity clinical information while incorporating, gathering, handling, examining, and removing information comprises a difficult assignment (M. Rathore et al., 2017).

P. Kaur et al. (2019) have used different ML models like KNN, Decision Tree, SVM, Random Forest, etc. over freely available datasets for monitoring the patients at remote geographical locations. The authors have proposed a framework that would help in disease prediction. S.K. Mohan et al. (2019) presented a hybrid prediction model to predict cardiovascular disease using

Random Forest supervised machine learning using a linear model (HRFLM). This study is done using the UCI machine learning repository for a dataset.

H. Fouad et al. (2020) used iterative golden section optimized deep beliefneural network (IGDBN) using Matlabtool to analyze and predict patient's health based on previous health records. The authors used Matthews correlation co-efficient, precision, accuracy and other parameters to find out the efficiency of their method. Kwok Tai Chui et al. (2017) reviewed many studies in which machine learning played an important role in diagnosing the disease in a smart environment. The authors discussed various ML models that are very popular in the fields of disease prediction like Heart related diseases, type 2 diabetes, Alzheimer Disease and Other Forms of Dementia, etc.

S.K. Lakshmanaprabu et al. (2019) collected real-time data of more than 100 thousand people every day by monitoring patients having heart, lungs, kidney and liver disorders and storing it in a database. After that, the authors have used Hadoop, MapReduce and Machine l Learning classifiers to access and analyze the huge IoT dataset. To classify the dataset, authors have used RFC (Random Forest Classifier). Precision of this classifier is 94.23% and 89.99% recall. These parameters help in measuring the performance of the model used.

Muhammad Attique Khan et al. (2020) researched Gastrointestinal Diseases. Authors have also focused on the artificial intelligence techniques that can be used for pathology and WCE by analyzing medical images and diagnosing the infected areas in the images. 6000 RGB images of WCE modularity are used as a dataset. A pre-trained DL model trains the dataset and then cubical SVM is used to classify the dataset based on respective features. Authors have used Matlab as a platform to perform the classification and get 96.50% accuracy. Other classifiers like LSVM (Linear SVM), QSVM (Quadratic SVM), Co-SVM (Coarse SVM), FKNN (Fine KNN), EBT (Ensemble Boosted Tree), and DT (Decision Tree) are also used but CSVM outperforms other classifiers.

Jun Qi et al. (2020) presented their study on some data fission techniques using machine learning algorithms. This technique helps in recalling and measuring physical activities by the patients in an IoT-enabled environment. The authors described different sensors that can be used to measure physical activities and these activities can be detected by analyzing data collected by the sensor used. ML models like SVM, RF, KNN), Naive Bayes (NB), etc. are used for physical activity recognition purposes. Jun Qi et al. (2018) also presented a systematic review of the healthcare physical activity monitoring system. The author presented architecture as Physical Activity Recognition and Monitoring (PRAM) to detect physical activities like walking, jogging, driving, sitting, swimming, laying, etc.

Musaed Alhussein et al. (2018) detected the efficiency of the voice pathology system on a healthcare system using deep learning technique. Authors have used CNN (Convolutional Neural Network) to analyze the pre-processed voice signals. For this detection purpose 'Saarbrucken voice disorder' dataset is used. Applying CNN model on the voice pathology system gives an accuracy around 97.5%.

3. IoT in Healthcare

IoT in the medical field has introduced a new word Internet of Medical Things (IoMT). It is an extraordinary class of IoT where the clinical gadgets speak with one another for sharing delicate information (R.M. Swarnapriya et al., 2020). IoT empowered sensor devices have made remote observation of patients in the medical services area feasible, helps to keep patients safe and sound and helps doctors to provide standout care to the patients. Similarly, it has increased patients' commitment and fulfillment because co-operations with respective doctors is much easier now. In addition to this, remote observing helps patients to have good and homely care at home only rather than a medical clinic. Additionally, IoT helps in significantly minimizing the medical care costs.

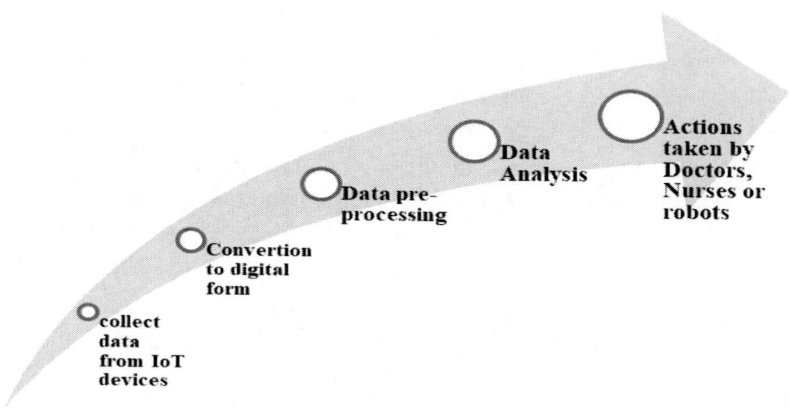

Figure 3. IoMT Working Steps.

IoMT working process is explained in the following steps (Figure 3)

- First step: Different healthcare devices like monitor screens, actuators, cameras, sensors, etc. are connected with the internet. These devices are used to gather data and arrange it collectively with the help of internet.
- Second step: This raw data collected by different IoT devices is in analog form, which is digitalized for further data processing activities.
- Third step: This digital data have to go from multiple data pre-processing steps like data cleaning, normalizing, standardizing, etc. After all data pre-processing steps, data is passed to the data centers or clouds for analysis purpose.
- Fourth step: In this step, collected pre-processed data is analyzed using different statistical and machine learning algorithms.
- Fifth step: This analysis output is sent to doctors, healthcare providers (nurses, etc.), or robots, which can take respective actions based on the insights provided by the data analysis step.

Healthcare system is a system that is created by the combined efforts of healthcare service providers (doctors, nurses, etc.), patients, healthcare insurance providers, etc. There are multiple applications of IoT in the domain of healthcare, which are explained below:

- **Healthcare Monitoring:** IoT devices help doctors and nurses to monitor remote patients. It also helps patients to have a check on themselves. . Different wearable devices or IoT sensors help to monitor health metrics like blood pressure, pulse rate, body temperature, glucose monitoring, and many more.
  IoT devices help **Parkinson's patients** to live their own lives in their own homes. IoT devices can also be used to monitor the mood of **patients of depression**. **Asthma patients** can be monitored with the help of sensor devices; more over, connected inhalers help asthma patients to carry their inhalers with them always. In case they forget to carry their inhalers on their way out from home, patients get alerts in the smart device.
- **Surgeries:** To collect data from inside of the human body, different **ingestible sensors** can also be used. These devices can be swallowed by a person easily moreover these devices get dissolved or get

disposed from the human body without doing any harm to it. These type of devices are generally used for pH or stomach monitoring for further surgeries.

By sending **little IoT robots** inside a human body, healthcare specialists can perform those surgeries also, that would be hard to oversee utilizing human hands. Simultaneously, mechanical medical procedures performed by little IoT gadgets can help to reduce deep cuts and stitches during medical procedure, which further helps in less obtrusive interaction as well as speedy recuperating for patients.

Gadgets to be used during surgery need to be sufficiently little as well as solid enough so that they can perform medical procedures without any disturbance. These little IoT gadgets must have the option to decipher tough medical scenarios while being inside human bodies so that they can reach a correct conclusion like, what steps should be taken throughout a medical procedure. However, small IoT robotic devices are as of now, being utilized for a medical procedure, showing that these difficulties can be sufficiently tended to.

- **Disease Prediction:** In the healthcare industry, different IoT sensor devices are used to collect perceptive data that can decide the life or death of a human being. This data helps in analyzing past records of the patients, which further becomes handy in predicting diseases in the future. So, developing or using correct ML algorithm for the respective scenario is a high priority subject in the healthcare industry. Also, for disease prediction, one can use advanced AI biosensors (Xiaofeng Jin et al., 2020).

The advantages of using IoT in the healthcare systems are shown in Figure 4. Though, every advanced technique comes with a price, there are some disadvantages. Security is one of the major concern

- **Security:** Security is an important concern in IoMT. In the Healthcare systems, enormous IoT devices are being used for gathering numerous measures of information. The utilization of IoMT builds huge volumes of unstructured data. A lot of confidential data of patients is present over the network. This data is needed to be handled with care. This kind of information can be used for any criminal activity if goes into the wrong hands. (Aidan Fuller et al., 2020)
- **Costly infrastructure:** To create a full-fledged setup for IoMT requires a huge amount of investment which is not possible for every

healthcare-providing organization. Though developed countries are successful to cross these bars but in developing and underdeveloped countries, this could be quite a nightmare.

- **Obsolete infrastructure:** Existing setup of healthcare industries is very obsolete. Some of them may not have IT setup also. So to create an IoMT environment in healthcare industries, one needs to work from the root to the leaves of a healthcare industry tree.

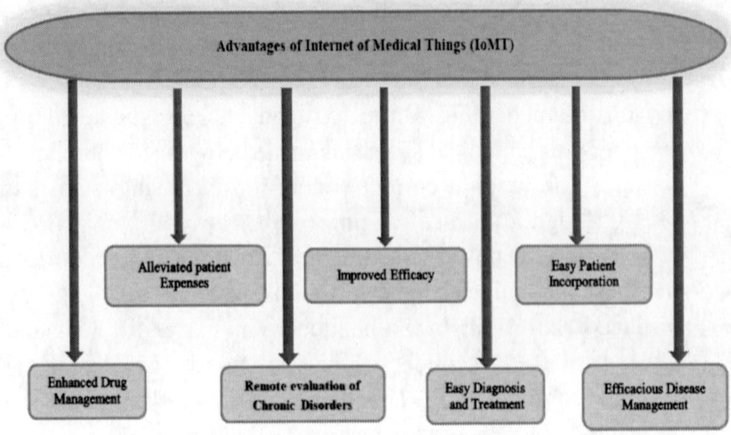

Figure 4. Advantages of IoMT.

3.1 Machine Learning in IoMT

Machine Learning (ML) is the most revolutionary innovation that has commanded the notice of researchers and industrial professionals and is relied upon to develop soon. Indeed, Machine Learning prepares the Internet of Things (IoT) to uphold communication among different devices without human associations. ML techniques are being used in multiple domains of IoT like healthcare, agriculture, smart homes, smart transportation, energy domain, data security, etc. (IkramUd Din et al., 2019).

Since the current COVID-19 situation, there has surfaced a requirement of a technology that can detect disease, analyse it and help in decision making. These decision-making technologies may help the healthcare providers by not being in direct physical contact with the patient. This kind of technology can only be developed with the integration of IoT and Machine Learning. (RajuVaishya et al., 2020)

A huge amount of heterogeneous data is collected from IoMT network, as shown in Figure 5. In IoMT we collect data from different sensors that are used in the following application areas of healthcare:

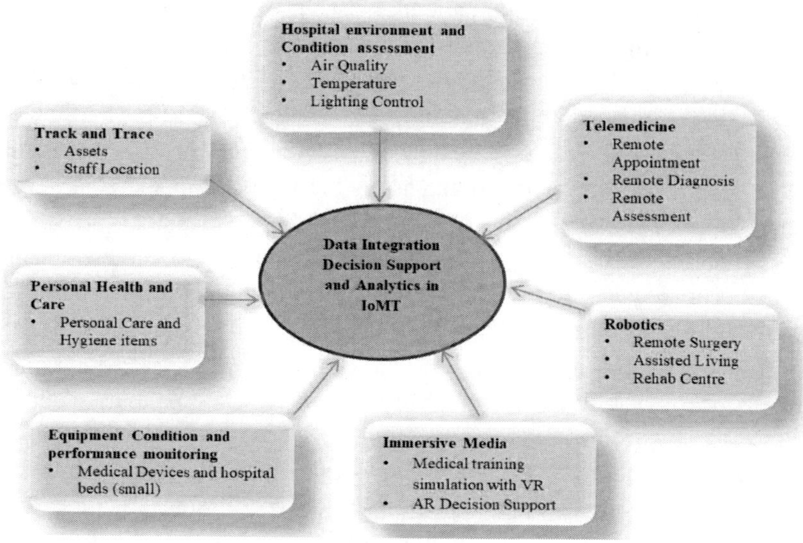

Figure 5. Data Integration and Analytics in IoMT.

- **Hospital Environment and Condition Assessment Sensors:** These sensors help to collect environmental data like air quality, surroundings temperature and lighting control, etc.
- **Telemedicine:** Telemedicine is a technique that uses the telephonic verbal connection between the physician and the patient. This is a very successful practice for remote patients monitoring. Patients can book their appointments using IoT devices and doctors can use same to diagnose the patient from different locations.
- **Robotics:** Nowadays, robots are also in common use for the living assistance of patients who are not capable of handling themselves. These are also used in rehab centers to have an eye on serious patients. Moreover, tiny robots are also very helpful during surgeries. These tiny robots help to operate in those areas where human hands are not effective.
- **Immersive Media:** Media is very effective in providing medical training under the simulation with the help of virtual reality.

- **Equipment Condition and performance monitoring:** In hi-tech medical hospitals, small hospital beds having internet controlled medical devices are used.
- **Personal Healthcare:** Many dieticians, physicians have a regular check on their regular patients regarding their personal healthcare on a daily basis and it is not possible for the patients also to visit one's dietician or physician on a regular basis. That's why today we use IoT to keep up and track in both ways.
- **Track and Trace:** In healthcare environment, it is very necessary to keep track of their staff and assets for any kind of emergency case.

Data collected from the above applications of IoT in healthcare is necessary to be analyzed to get insights. Data collected from different IoT healthcare devices are integrated and then analyzed to reach any decision. These decisions are made using different AI techniques and ML is one of them. Machine learning and Deep learning can be used to diagnose, analyze, and rectify any healthcare problem within the shortest time possible (S. Durga et al., 2019). However, one should know which algorithm will be applicable and when it should be applied. Description of different Healthcare IoT activities which use machine learning techniques to achieve their respective goals is depicted in Table 1.

Table 1. Machine learning techniques used in IoMT

S. No.	IoMT activity	Machine Learning Techniques	References
1.	Heart Disease Prediction	Hybrid Random Forest with linear model	S.K. Mohan et al. (2019)
2.	Monitoring System	Random Forest (RF)	P. Kaur et al. (2019)
3.	Disease Analysis	Random Forest Classifier	S.K. Lakshmanaprabu et al. (2019)
4.	Gastrointestinal Diseases Analysis	Support Vector Machine (SVM)	Muhammad Attique Khan et al. (2020)
5.	Physical Activity recognition	SVM, KNN, Bayes, RF	Jun Qi et al. (2020)
6.	Voice Pathology	CNN	MusaedAlhussein et al. (2018)
7.	Ophthalmology	DL	Ji-Peng Olivia Li et al. (2021)
8.	Intrusion Detection in IoMT	DNN, KNN, Naive Bayes, RF, SVM	SwarnaPriya R.M. et al. (2020)
S. No.	IoMT activity	Machine Learning Techniques	References

9.	Patient Health Analysis	Deep Belief Neural Network (DBNN)	H. Fouad et al. (2020)
10.	Encryption on ECG data	Supervised machine learning i.e., SVM	Han Qiu et al. (2020)
11.	Predicting Labour Complications Based on Stress	SVM, KNN, Naive Bayes (NB), Decision Tree (DT)	V. Madhusri et al. (2019)
12.	Clinical Analysis	Noval C 4.5 DT	Shin-Jye Lee et al. (2018)
13.	Personalized Smart Health Application	TESLA, Hidden Markov Model (HMM), Bayesian network, ANN	Jaganathan Venkatesh et al. (2018)
14.	Parkinson's disease affected patient's monitoring	K-means clustering	DebanjanBorthakur et al. (2018)
15.	Elderly people's fall detection system	Decision Tree	Diana Yacchirema et al. (2018)
16.	War Soldier's health monitoring	K-means, unsupervised clustering technique	AashayGondalia et al. (2018)
17.	Stress Detection	LR, SVM, Naive Bayes	Purnendu Shekhar Pandey (2017)

4. Bibliometric Analysis

Bibliometric analysis is done over Web of Sciences and Scopus datasets. These datasets are explored and used to export a large number of papers for study. These papers are exported on the basis of some keywords used for searching, which are shown in Table 2. Duplicates found in the exported database of papers are also removed. These papers are further filtered out based on different constrained applied by the author.

Table 2. Different datasets used for analysis

S. No.	Dataset	Keyword set for searching	#papers found	Duplicates found	Actual results
1.	WOS	TOPIC: (IoT) AND TOPIC: (Machine Learning) AND TOPIC: (Healthcare) Timespan: 2018-2021.	401	0	401
2.	Scopus	Title, abstract, keywords: "IoT" AND "Machine Learning" AND "Healthcare" Timespan: 2018-2021.	506	3	503

In the Scopus dataset, 506 documents were exported and after the removal of duplicates, we found 503 results. 31 documents are filtered out on the basis of most cited (more than 25 citations) documents which are clustered on the basis of their connectivity strength. 27 such types of clusters are formed. Overlays visualization of these clusters is shown in Figure 6.

In WoS data, there were no duplicates found and as a result, 401 papers are used for analysis. 20 documents are filtered out on the basis of most cited (more than 25 citations) documents which are clustered on the basis of their connectivity strength. 18 such types of clusters are formed. Overlays visualization of these clusters is shown in Figure 7.

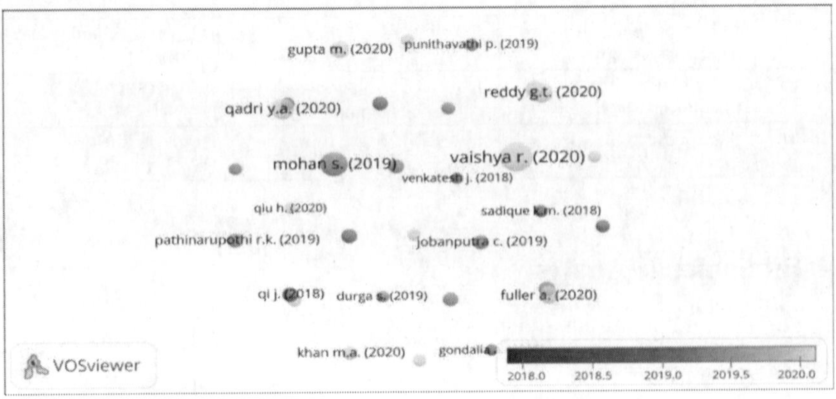

Figure 6. Overlay Visualization of Scopus Indexed Documents.

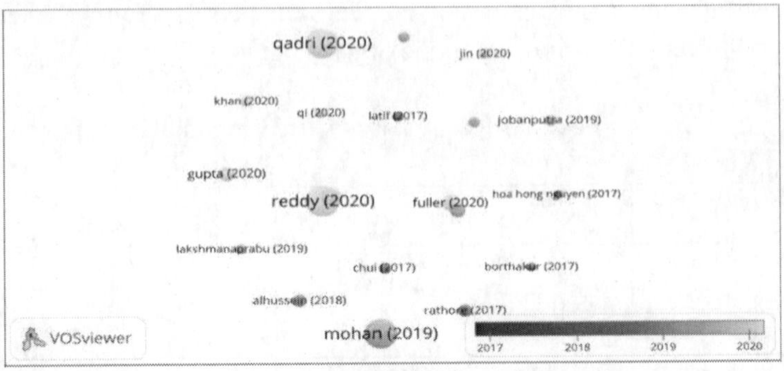

Figure 7. Overlay Visualization of WoS Indexed Documents.

Organization based bibliometric analysis is also done in this study. Some constraints are set initially to precede further for organizational analysis with respect to both datasets i.e., Scopus as well as Web of Sciences. For the Scopus dataset, we have considered only those studies for analysis in which there are a most 15 organizations are involved in the study. Also, a minimum number of documents with respect to an organization must be at least 3, and a minimum number of citations of an organization must be atleast 7 are some of the initial constraints. As a result, 5 out of 1280 organizations fit in the description. Among which 'Alagappa University, India' gave highest citations i.e., 148 citations. These five organizations with their cited documents are shown in Table 3.

For the WoS dataset, we have considered only those studies for analysis in which there are atmost 7 organizations are involved in the study. Also, a minimum number of documents with respect to an organization must be atleast 5 and a minimum number of citations of an organization must be atleast 7 are some of the initial constraints. As a result, 11 out of 716 organizations fit in the description. Among which 'King Saud Univ. gave the highest citations i.e., 137 citations. The top five organizations with their cited documents are shown in Table 4.

Table 3. Organization-wise citation analysis on Scopus database

Organization	#Documents	#citations
Dept of Comp. Applications, Alagappa University, India	3	148
Universitatpolitecnica da valencia	4	28
Liverpool John Moores University, United Kingdom	3	26
Dept. of Cyber Security, Air university, Islamabad, Pakistan	4	22
Dept of Comp sci, Air University, Islamabad, Pakistan	3	13

Table 4. Organization-wise citation analysis on WoS database

Organization	#Documents	#citations
King Saud Univ.	18	137
Vellore Institute Techno	5	85
Natl. Univ. Comp & emerging sci	7	58
Qatar Univ.	5	52
Natl. Univ. Singapore	8	43

5. Methodology and Results Analysis

For this study "Heart Failure Prediction" dataset (DavideChicco et al., 2020) is used for the prediction. In this dataset, we have around 13 attributes. Jupyter notebook is used as a platform for the analysis of this dataset. Libraries of python like Matplotlib, SciLearn, Numpy are used. The methodology used for the working process is shown in Figure 8. This dataset was not balanced, so to balance the dataset we have used an imbalanced learn library of python. After the normalization of a dataset, we applied different Machine Learning Algorithms then compared their performance based on matrices like Accuracy, Recall, F1 score, and Precision. Different Machine learning algorithms like Linear Regression (LR), Decision Tree (DT), K- Nearest Neighbour (KNN), Random Forest (RF), Naive Bayes (NB), Support Vector Machine (SVM) are used for analysis.

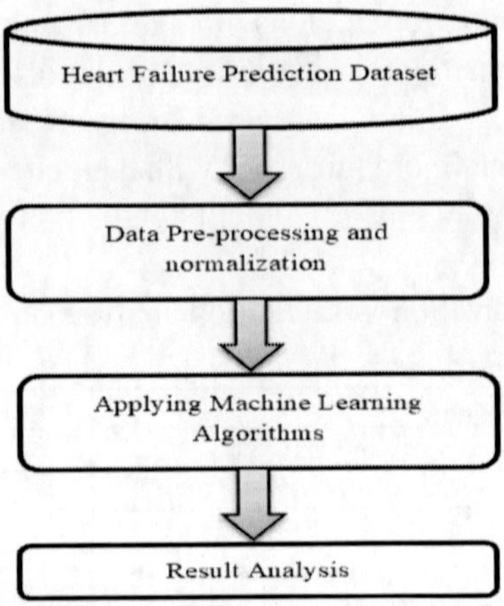

Figure 8. Process Flow.

Table 5. Comparative analysis of ML algorithms

Measures → / ↓ML Algorithm	Accuracy	Precision	Recall	F measure
Linear Regression	0.74	0.79	0.63	0.70
Naive Bayes	0.683	0.829	0.442	0.576
Decision Tree	0.74	0.765	0.675	0.717
Support Vector Machine	0.784	0.787	0.766	0.776
Random Forest	0.82	0.851	0.818	0.834
K- Nearest Neighbour	0.73	0.70	0.77	0.74

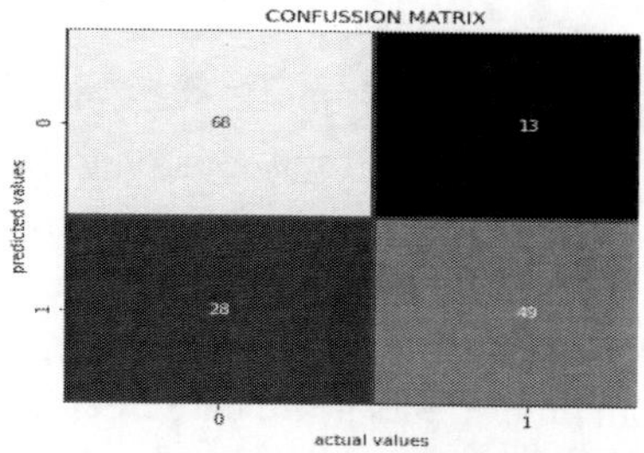

(a) Confusion matrix of LR

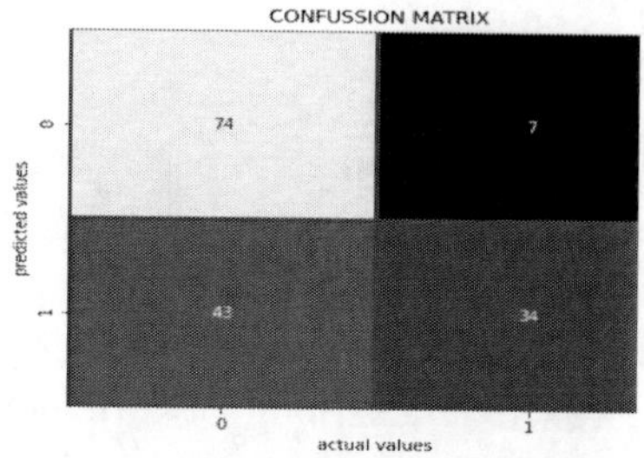

(b) Confusion matrix of NB

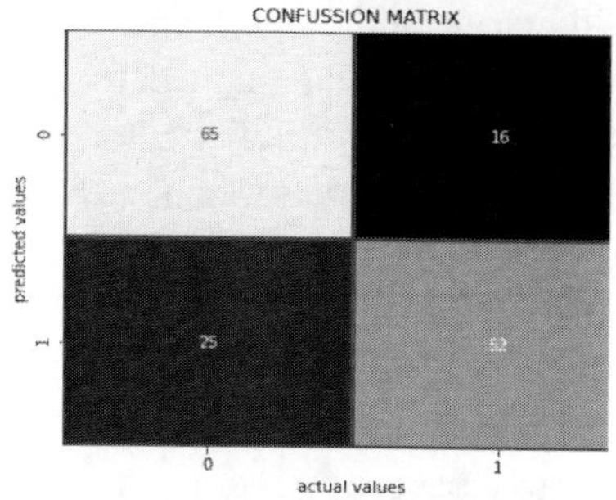

(c) Confusion matrix of DT

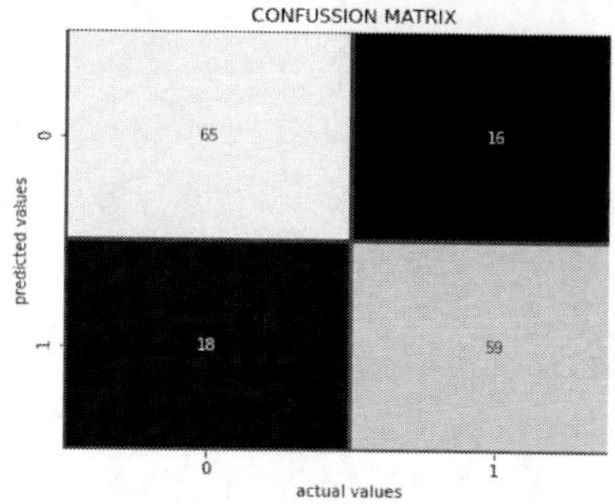

(c) Confusion matrix of SVM

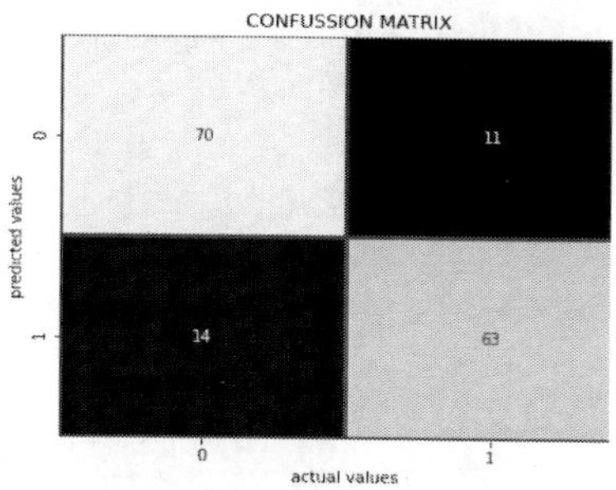

(e) Confusion matrix of RF

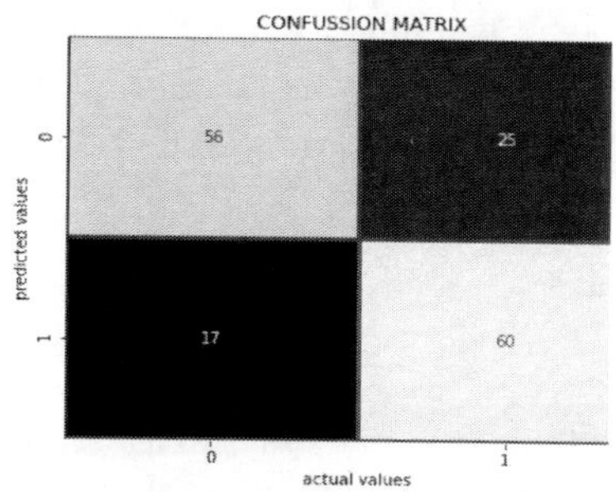

(d) Confusion matrix of KNN

Figure 9. Confusion Matrix of ML Algorithms.

As seen in the results, Random Forest has outperformed all other machine learning techniques. It attains an accuracy of 82%, which is much better than the accuracy of DT, which is 74%, accuracy of Linear Regression is given at 74%. Support vector Machine accuracy is given at 78.4%. K-nearest neighbour supervised machine learning technology is given at 73% and Naive Bayes accuracy is 68.3%.

Conclusion

IoT has become integral part of humans in everyday life in society across the globe. Integration of IoT and Machine Learning makes a powerful combination for the Healthcare sector. In the healthcare domain, technology plays an important role in its up-gradation. This study explains the role of IoT and Machine Learning in different domains of the healthcare sectors like disease prediction, remote patient monitoring, surgeries by tiny robots and biosensors to track and trace. This study presents an erudite literature review for an understanding of recent important work being done in this area.

Scopus and Web of Sciences datasets are used for bibliometric analysis for IoT-enabled healthcare environments using effective Machine Learning techniques. Bibliometric analysis helps to choose different studies and research works to gain a piece of valuable knowledge. Through bibliometric analysis, most active organizations are rated based on their work citations. "Heart Failure Dataset" is taken for analysis of different supervised Machine Learning techniques. The dataset is firstly pre-processed by eliminating duplicates from it and balancing the imbalanced data. After normalizing the data, six machine learning techniques are applied. Out of all ML techniques used, RF accuracy came out to be the best as 0.82, Precision as 0.85, recall as 0.81, and F1 measure as 0.834.

References

Abdulameer, Taisir Hasan, Abdullahi Abdu IBRAHIM, and Alaa Hamid Mohammed. 2020. "Design of Health Care Monitoring System Based on Internet of Thing (IOT)." In 2020 *4th International Symposium on Multidisciplinary Studies and Innovative Technologies (ISMSIT)*, 1–6. https://doi.org/10.1109/ ISMSIT50672.2020.9254291.

Aktas, Faruk, CelalCeken, and YunusEmreErdemli. 2018. "IoT-Based Healthcare Framework for Biomedical Applications." *Journal of Medical and Biological Engineering*, 38 (6): 966–79. https://doi.org/10.1007/s40846-017-0349-7.

Alhussein, Musaed, and Ghulam Muhammad. 2018. "Voice Pathology Detection Using Deep Learning on Mobile Healthcare Framework." *IEEE Access* 6: 41034–41. https://doi.org/10.1109/ACCESS.2018.2856238.

Borthakur, Debanjan, Harishchandra Dubey, Nicholas Constant, Leslie Mahler, and KunalMankodiya. 2017. "Smart Fog: Fog Computing Framework for Unsupervised Clustering Analytics in Wearable Internet of Things." In *2017 IEEE Global Conference on Signal and Information Processing (GlobalSIP)*, 472–76. https://doi.org/10.1109/GlobalSIP.2017.8308687.

Chicco, Davide, and Giuseppe Jurman. 2020. "Machine Learning Can Predict Survival of Patients with Heart Failure from Serum Creatinine and Ejection Fraction Alone." *BMC Medical Informatics and Decision Making*, 20 (1): 16. https://doi.org/10.1186/s12911-020-1023-5.

Chui, Kwok Tai, WadeeAlhalabi, Sally Shuk Han Pang, Patricia Ordóñez de Pablos, Ryan Wen Liu, and Mingbo Zhao. 2017. "Disease Diagnosis in Smart Healthcare: Innovation, Technologies and Applications." *Sustainability*, 9 (12): 2309. https://doi.org/10.3390/su9122309.

Din, IkramUd, Mohsen Guizani, Joel J. P. C. Rodrigues, Suhaidi Hassan, and Valery V. Korotaev. 2019. "Machine Learning in the Internet of Things: Designed Techniques for Smart Cities." *Future Generation Computer Systems*, 100 (November): 826–43. https://doi.org/10.1016/j.future.2019.04.017.

Durga, S., Rishabh Nag, and Esther Daniel. 2019. "Survey on Machine Learning and Deep Learning Algorithms Used in Internet of Things (IoT) Healthcare." In *2019 3rd International Conference on Computing Methodologies and Communication (ICCMC)*, 1018–22.https://doi.org/10.1109/ICCMC.2019.8819806.

Firouzi, Farshad, BaharFarahani, Mohamed Ibrahim, and KrishnenduChakrabarty. 2018. "Keynote Paper: From EDA to IoTEHealth: Promises, Challenges, and Solutions." *IEEE Transactions on Computer-Aided Design of Integrated Circuits and Systems*, 37 (12): 2965–78. https://doi.org/10.1109/TCAD.2018.2801227.

Fouad, H., Azza S. Hassanein, Ahmed M. Soliman, and Haytham Al-Feel. 2020. "Analyzing Patient Health Information Based on IoT Sensor with AI for Improving Patient Assistance in the Future Direction." *Measurement*, 159 (July): 107757. https://doi.org/10.1016/j.measurement.2020.107757.

Fuller, Aidan, Zhong Fan, Charles Day, and Chris Barlow. 2020. "Digital Twin: Enabling Technologies, Challenges and Open Research." *IEEE Access*, 8: 108952–71. https://doi.org/10.1109/ACCESS.2020.2998358.

Gondalia, Aashay, Dhruv Dixit, Shubham Parashar, Vijayanand Raghava, Animesh Sengupta, and Vergin Raja Sarobin. 2018. "IoT-Based Healthcare Monitoring System for War Soldiers Using Machine Learning." *Procedia Computer Science, International Conference on Robotics and Smart Manufacturing (RoSMa2018)*, 133 (January): 1005–13. https://doi.org/10.1016/j.procs.2018.07.075.

Gopal, Gayatri, Clemens Suter-Crazzolara, Luca Toldo, and Werner Eberhardt. 2019. "Digital Transformation in Healthcare – Architectures of Present and Future Information Technologies." *Clinical Chemistry and Laboratory Medicine (CCLM)*, 57 (3): 328–35. https://doi.org/10.1515/cclm-2018-0658.

Jin, Xiaofeng, Conghui Liu, TailinXu, Lei Su, and Xueji Zhang. 2020. "Artificial Intelligence Biosensors: Challenges and Prospects." *Biosensors and Bioelectronics*, 165 (October): 112412. https://doi.org/10.1016/j.bios.2020.112412.

Jobanputra, Charmi, Jatna Bavishi, and Nishant Doshi. 2019. "Human Activity Recognition: A Survey." Procedia Computer Science, The 16th International Conference on Mobile Systems and Pervasive Computing (MobiSPC 2019), The 14th International Conference on Future Networks and Communications (FNC-2019), *The 9th International Conference on Sustainable Energy Information Technology*, 155 (January): 698–703. https://doi.org/10.1016/j.procs.2019.08.100.

Kaur, Pavleen, Ravinder Kumar, and Munish Kumar. 2019. "A Healthcare Monitoring System Using Random Forest and Internet of Things (IoT)." *Multimedia Tools and Applications*, 78 (14): 19905–16. https://doi.org/10.1007/s11042-019-7327-8.

khan, Imran, Kamran Zeb, Asif Mahmood, Waqar Uddin, Muhammad Adil Khan, Saif-ul-Islam, and Hee Je Kim. 2019. "Healthcare Monitoring System and Transforming Monitored Data into Real Time Clinical Feedback Based on IoT Using Raspberry Pi." In *2019 2nd International Conference on Computing, Mathematics and Engineering Technologies (ICoMET)*, 1–6.https://doi.org/10.1109/ ICOMET.2019.8673393.

Khan, Muhammad Attique, Seifedine Kadry, Majed Alhaisoni, Yunyoung Nam, Yudong Zhang, Venkatesan Rajinikanth, and Muhammad Shahzad Sarfraz. 2020. "Computer-Aided Gastrointestinal Diseases Analysis From Wireless Capsule Endoscopy: A Framework of Best Features Selection." *IEEE Access*, 8: 132850–59. https://doi.org/10.1109/ACCESS.2020.3010448.

Lakshmanaprabu, S. K., K. Shankar, M. Ilayaraja, Abdul Wahid Nasir, V. Vijayakumar, and Naveen Chilamkurti. 2019. "Random Forest for Big Data Classification in the Internet of Things Using Optimal Features." *International Journal of Machine Learning and Cybernetics*, 10 (10): 2609–18. https://doi.org/10.1007/s13042-018-00916-z.

Lee, Shin-Jye, ZhaozhaoXu, Tong Li, and Yun Yang. 2018. "A Novel Bagging C4.5 Algorithm Based on Wrapper Feature Selection for Supporting Wise Clinical Decision Making." *Journal of Biomedical Informatics*, 78 (February): 144–55. https://doi.org/10.1016/j.jbi.2017.11.005.

Li, Ji-Peng Olivia, Hanruo Liu, Darren S. J. Ting, Sohee Jeon, R. V. Paul Chan, Judy E. Kim, Dawn A. Sim, et al. 2021. "Digital Technology, Tele-Medicine and Artificial Intelligence in Ophthalmology: A Global Perspective." *Progress in Retinal and Eye Research*, 82 (May): 100900. https://doi.org/10.1016/j.preteyeres.2020.100900.

Madhusri, V., G. Kesavkrishna, Ramalatha Marimuthu, and Sathyanarayanan R. 2019. "Performance Comparison of Machine Learning Algorithms to Predict Labor Complications and Birth Defects Based On Stress." In *2019 IEEE 10th International Conference on Awareness Science and Technology (ICAST)*, 1–5. https://doi.org/10.1109/ICAwST.2019.8923370.

Majumdar, Arun K. 2019. "Chapter 8 - Free-Space Optical Communications: Role and Integration With the Internet of Things." In *Optical Wireless Communications for Broadband Global Internet Connectivity*, edited by Arun K. Majumdar, 245–58.Elsevier.https://doi.org/10.1016/B978-0-12-813365-1.00008-4.

Mazhar, Rathore M, Paul Anand, Ahmad Awais, Anisetti Marco, and Jeon Gwanggil. 2017. "Hadoop-Based Intelligent Care System (HICS)." *ACM Transactions on Internet Technology (TOIT)*, November. https://doi.org/10.1145/3108936.

Mohan, Senthilkumar, Chandrasegar Thirumalai, and Gautam Srivastava. 2019. "Effective Heart Disease Prediction Using Hybrid Machine Learning Techniques." *IEEE Access*, 7: 81542–54. https://doi.org/10.1109/ACCESS.2019.2923707.

Nguyen, Hoa Hong, FarhaanMirza, M. AsifNaeem, and Minh Nguyen. 2017. "A Review on IoT Healthcare Monitoring Applications and a Vision for Transforming Sensor Data into Real-Time Clinical Feedback." In *2017 IEEE 21st International Conference on Computer Supported Cooperative Work in Design (CSCWD)*, 257–62. https://doi.org/10.1109/CSCWD.2017.8066704.

Pandey, PurnenduShekhar. 2017. "Machine Learning and IoT for Prediction and Detection of Stress." In *2017 17th International Conference on Computational Science and Its Applications (ICCSA)*, 1–5. https://doi.org/10.1109/ ICCSA.2017.8000018.

Pantelopoulos, Ros, and Nikolaos G. Bourbakis. 2010. "A Survey on Wearable Sensor-Based Systems for Health Monitoring and Prognosis." *IEEE Transactions on Systems, MAN, and Cybernetics-Part C: Applications and Reviews.*

Pathinarupothi, Rahul Krishnan, P Durga, and Ekanath Srihari Rangan. 2019. "IoT-Based Smart Edge for Global Health: Remote Monitoring With Severity Detection and Alerts Transmission." *IEEE Internet of Things Journal*, 6 (2): 2449–62. https://doi.org/10.1109/JIOT.2018.2870068.

Qadri, Yazdan Ahmad, Ali Nauman, Yousaf Bin Zikria, Athanasios V. Vasilakos, and Sung Won Kim. 2020. "The Future of Healthcare Internet of Things: A Survey of Emerging Technologies." *IEEE Communications Surveys Tutorials*, 22 (2): 1121–67. https://doi.org/10.1109/COMST.2020.2973314.

Qi, Jun, Po Yang, Atif Waraich, Zhikun Deng, Youbing Zhao, and Yun Yang. 2018. "Examining Sensor-Based Physical Activity Recognition and Monitoring for Healthcare Using Internet of Things: A Systematic Review." *Journal of Biomedical Informatics*, 87 (November): 138–53. https://doi.org/10.1016/j.jbi.2018.09.002.

Qi, Jun, Po Yang, Lee Newcombe, XiyangPeng, Yun Yang, and Zhong Zhao. 2020. "An Overview of Data Fusion Techniques for Internet of Things Enabled Physical Activity Recognition and Measure." *Information Fusion*, 55 (March): 269–80. https://doi.org/10.1016/j.inffus.2019.09.002.

Qiu, Han, MeikangQiu, and Zhihui Lu. 2020. "Selective Encryption on ECG Data in Body Sensor Network Based on Supervised Machine Learning." *Information Fusion*, 55 (March): 59–67. https://doi.org/10.1016/j.inffus.2019.07.012.

R.m., SwarnaPriya, Praveen Kumar Reddy Maddikunta, Parimala M., Srinivas Koppu, Thippa Reddy Gadekallu, Chiranji Lal Chowdhary, and MamounAlazab. 2020. "An Effective Feature Engineering for DNN Using Hybrid PCA-GWO for Intrusion Detection in IoMT Architecture." *Computer Communications*, 160 (July): 139–49. https://doi.org/10.1016/j.comcom.2020.05.048.

Sethi, Pallavi, and Smruti R. Sarangi. 2017. "Internet of Things: Architectures, Protocols, and Applications." *Journal of Electrical and Computer Engineering*, 2017 (January): e9324035. https://doi.org/10.1155/2017/9324035.

Singh, Kiran Jot, and Divneet Singh Kapoor. 2017. "Create Your Own Internet of Things: A Survey of IoT Platforms." *IEEE Consumer Electronics Magazine*, 6 (2): 57–68. https://doi.org/10.1109/MCE.2016.2640718.

Vaishya, Raju, Mohd Javaid, Ibrahim Haleem Khan, and Abid Haleem. 2020. "Artificial Intelligence (AI) Applications for COVID-19 Pandemic." *Diabetes & Metabolic Syndrome: Clinical Research & Reviews*, 14 (4): 337–39. https://doi.org/10.1016/j.dsx.2020.04.012.

Venkatesh, Jaganathan, Baris Aksanli, Christine S. Chan, Alper Sinan Akyurek, and Tajana Simunic Rosing. 2018. "Modular and Personalized Smart Health Application Design in a Smart City Environment." *IEEE Internet of Things Journal*, 5 (2): 614–23. https://doi.org/10.1109/JIOT.2017.2712558.

Yacchirema, Diana, Jara Suárez de Puga, Carlos Palau, and Manuel Esteve. 2018. "Fall Detection System for Elderly People Using IoT and Big Data." *Procedia Computer Science*, *The 9th International Conference on Ambient Systems, Networks and Technologies (ANT 2018)/The 8th International Conference on Sustainable Energy Information Technology (SEIT-2018)/Affiliated Workshops*, 130 (January): 603–10. https://doi.org/10.1016/j.procs.2018.04.110.

Chapter 5

AI, IoT and Wearable Technology for Smart Health Care

M. Deepika[1,*] and D. Karthika[2]

[1]Assistant Professor, Department of Computer Science, B. S.Abdur Rahman Crescent Institute of Science and Technology, Chennai, Tamil Nadu

[2]Assistant Professor, Department of Computer Science, SDNB Vaishnav College for Women, Chennai, Tamil Nadu

Abstract

Health care is no longer an isolated industry unaffected by technological advances. Technology drives health care more than any other factor, and it will continue to do so in a remarkable manner in the future. Smart Wearables, IoT, Big Data, Cloud computing, and other cutting-edge technologies have transformed traditional health care into smart health care. In recent years, technology has enabled us to keep a close eye on our health. From bracelets that count steps and heart rate to body fat scales and blood pressure monitors, wearable technology has revolutionized our biology. In the following chapter, we discuss smart health care technologies, which have given the health care industry a new "smartness." Wearable technology can also be used to track lifestyle choices and improve personal health management. Consider the most important AI and IoT applications in the health care sector. In addition, many machine learning approaches can be applied to develop excellent decision support for health care applications.

*Corresponding Author's Email: deepika.rbp@gmail.com.

In: AI-Enabled IoT for Smart Health Care Systems
Editors: Tawseef Ayoub Shaikh, Tabasum Rasool and Mohammed Wasid
ISBN: 978-1-68507-977-2

Keywords: health care, smart wearables, artificial intelligence, big data, internet of things (IoT), smart health care

1. Introduction

The purpose of this section is to discuss intelligent health technologies that are changing the health care industry. Furthermore, it allows users to utilize portable technology to track their lifestyles and provide tools for better personal health management. Wearable devices are also available. Learn more about AI and IoT applications in health care. Health care decision support is being improved through the application of machine-learning algorithms. A hospital-centered health care system has been transformed into a patient-centered system thanks to technological advancements [2, 3]. Modern telecommunications technologies further enable clinical data to be transmitted to health centers in remote locations. Well-being wearables have been around for a long time. Computerized cardiac aids marked the start of the digital era in the late 1980s, coming about in an otherwise unused category of medical equipment. Wearable devices have advanced and learned to perform a wide range of tasks in various ways since that time. Smart sensors, artificial intelligence, and machine learning technologies are now actively being utilized in wearable devices.

1.1. Remote Patient Monitoring

Constant illnesses started in their early stages and progressed to regular schedules for well-being and life, as well as managing emergencies. Smart wearables have developed in the health care industry. In the US industry, these gadgets are expected to save over $200 billion over the next five years for the US industry. Approximately 180 billion dollars is expected to be spent worldwide on shrewd wearable devices by 2025. With the use of savvy sensors, fake insights, and machine learning, wearable gadgets are currently being delivered.

Although the Internet of Things did not expand freedom as it was meant to, it has also increased people's ability to interact with the outside world. IoT has become a key supporter of worldwide communication with the help of future conventions and calculations. Various devices, remote sensors, and home gadgets can be connected to the Web [4]. IoT is used in agriculture [5,

6], in vehicles [6, 7], in houses [8, 9], and restorative care. Because of its advantages of being more precise, cheaper, and able to anticipate future events, the Web of Things is gaining popularity. The fast IoT insurgency has picked up more understanding of computer programs and apps as a result of advances in portable and computer innovation, straightforward remote access, and a more advanced economy [11].

An implant or wearable sensor is used in restorative applications to obtain physiological data from the body (e.g., temperature, weight rate, ECG, EEG) of the patient. Data such as temperature, humidity, date, and time can be saved naturally. These data allow us to draw accurate and reliable conclusions about the health status of the patient. A high level of information capacity and accessibility is especially needed within the IoT framework since huge amounts of information are gathered from many sources (sensors, mobile phones, mail, programs, and applications). Detection devices provide information to doctors, professionals, and authorized individuals. This information can be shared with health care experts via cloud/server, allowing for quick diagnosis and, if necessary, treatment.

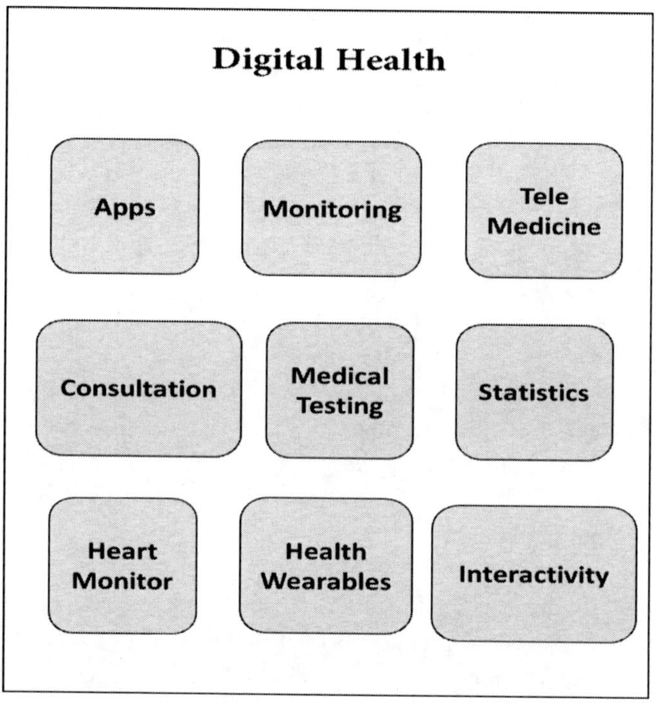

Figure 1. Health care Technologies.

To ensure efficient and secure transmission, communication between clients, patients, and the communication module will be maintained. Health care specialists utilize the majority of IoT frameworks to control patients, display information, and secure [12]. During the creation of an IoT system, the protection of quality-of-service networks is an essential issue, which involves protection, security, fetch, unwavering quality, and information-sharing accessibility.

Many nations have untapped innovation and laws to expand their businesses in health care frameworks. Therefore, the current investigation into wellness commerce has become an even more pertinent subject to look into. To clarify the current state of cutting-edge IoT wellbeing frameworks research and to assess its capabilities for innovation, administration, and applications, this chapter is written.

2. Artificial Intelligence and IoT in Health Care

- As AI and IoT are integrated with health care, operational efficiency is expected to increase. For the keen, successful application of AI calculations in IoT gadgets (modeling, forecasting), the following (collection), observing (investigation), and controlling (optimization) phases are essential. By working together, they can reduce the administrative burden on health care workers. Rehabilitation personnel will be able to spend more time with patients with improved clinical forms, and health care delivery will shift to a more patient-centered approach.
- As a result, the following AI-enabled IoT applications are most important:
- Inventory management, medical workers, and patients are all tracked.
- Chronic illness management
- The administration of drugs
- Emergency department wait times are halved.
- Monitoring health

AI and IoT are expected to improve operational effectiveness in health care. A smart, successful application of AI calculations in IoT gadgets (modeling, forecasting) involves following (collecting), checking (investigating), and controlling (optimizing). They work together to ease the regulatory burden on the health care workforce. With progressed clinical forms, the therapeutic workforce will have more time to spend with patients, while health care conveyance will shift to a more patient-centered approach. Medical applications can benefit from IoT and cloud computing through restorative applications. In addition, the document explains how information from sensors and medical equipment can be exchanged with the specific health care system. A health care topology is formed by partitioned IoT systems and networks that are always interconnected. In the past few years, there have been a few notable changes to the health care framework [15-17]. The connected activities within the arranged wellbeing application must be characterized when developing an IoT-based health care framework for real-time understanding monitoring. The success of an IoT framework depends on how well its requirements are met by health care providers. The topology must follow restorative rules and symptomatic stages since every condition requires an individual therapeutic action method.

3. Wearables and IoT Disrupting Health Care

Internet of Things (IoT) today defines many things, including how we manage and automate our living environment, how we shop, how we receive health care, and more.

As depicted in Figure 2, IoT and wearable's have resulted from significant corporate and societal changes, as well as from a variety of driving forces. A new age of advanced technology and associated commerce has dawned with wearables. In this age, people and companies collaborate in new and deeper ways. Contraptions communicate with other gadgets, and clients can choose what they need and require without regard to physical requirements. Coordination, setup, analysis, and administration systems, as well as continuous communication and arrangement, not just made the business successful, but additionally made it more effective than ever. Modern civilization has gained from it in various ways. Fashionables have the potential to transform business operations and models, as well as administration methods, while generating unused value, enhancing productivity, and paving the way for better ways to create income and provide better value to clients.

In the pharmaceutical and health care industries, wearables open up a world of possibilities. If conventional wearable restorative hardware is linked to the web, it may collect vital information that can save lives. As well, they offer additional information about any illness's physiological or mental symptoms. The internet of things enables further care, which was a science fiction concept, to become a reality. In a nutshell, IoT lets patients control their treatment and track the progress of their treatment using wearable devices connected to the internet [18].

4. The Next Decade is IoT's Decade

The next ten years or more are likely to see an upsurge in disease treatment and determination. Wearable gadgets in IoT provide companies, sponsors, clinicians, and patients with modern data and information. IoT gadgets provide therapeutic, pharmaceutical, and life-science companies with valuable information that helps them make informed decisions and compete more effectively. The advancement of IoT, as well through advancement of IoT, as well as its continued collaboration with pharmaceutical and restorative businesses, progress will be made towards real-time disease observation and treatment.

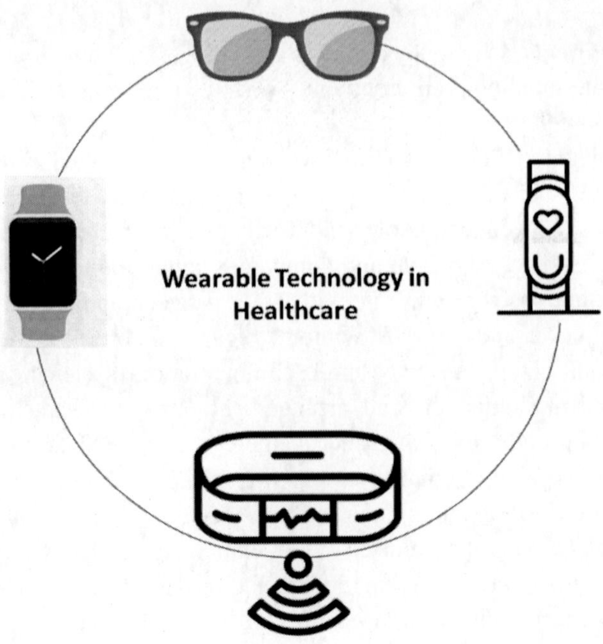

Figure 2. Wearable Technologies in Health care.

4.1. Glucose Trackers

One in eleven people worldwide has diabetes. Moreover, 46 percent of diabetics don't conclude. As of now, there are a handful of devices that can help in supplying stimuli to the body and observing glucose levels. Diabetes wearables include continuous glucose monitoring and automated glucose delivery systems. Dexcom and EverSense are the most well-known persistent glucose screens. EverSense's FDA-approved glucose monitor measures and records glucose levels for up to 90 days. Patients with type 1 diabetes can now take control of their diabetes autonomously thanks to a joint therapeutic wear device. This device permits patients with type 1 diabetes to manage their condition independently.

4.2. Wearables for Heart Attacks

The two most well-known nonstop glucose monitors are Dexcom and Ever Sense. A continuous glucose monitor that's FDA-approved, EverSense uses an embedded sensor to continuously monitor glucose levels for up to 90 days. Cardiovascular defibrillators can benefit patients with sporadic heartbeats. These devices monitor irregular heartbeats with little drums on the chest. You can mimic a moderate pulse when yours becomes too moderate. Studies have shown that implantable defibrillators can help predict sudden death in patients suffering from fibrillation or tachycardia.

4.3. Protection against Concussion

Sports-related concussions and wounds are protected by wearing a wearable gadget around the neck [20-21]. As the brain develops inside the skull, clogs form. A brain injury caused by such a capable development may lead to anatomical changes within the brain. Q-Collars work by tightening the jawbone within the neck to secure the brain within the cranium by using the body's physiology. Increased blood flow in the brain reduces the risk of developing cognitive diseases. Not only are capable blows to the head dangerous. Known as strikes, little, tedious blows can affect the brain and cause basic anomalies. Wearable Q-Collars protect against intemperate brain development. A ruckus is not only caused by effective blows to the head. An auxiliary brain anomaly can be caused by small, monotonous blows known as strikes. Intemperate brain development can be prevented with a Q-Collar.

4.4. Sensors for Stroke Patients

Sensors that measure muscle movement can be used to assist stroke patients and prosthesis patients in recovering from their injuries. By measuring muscle movement, EMG sensors aid in muscle testing and strengthening. Non-invasive and remote, these sensors can also evaluate the condition of nerves and muscles in damaged tissue.

4.5. Asthma Monitoring

When asthmatic individuals are in an attack, they will not realize it is happening until it has progressed. In most cases, the environment is unsafe and unworthy. Although treatment can help patients fight the attack, they have been affected and their vitality has been drained by the sensitivity. The wearable innovation for asthma observation can foresee asthma attacks, recently an understanding even recognizes the symptoms of the disease. In the current state of affairs, the medicine is whipped off and used to relieve the effects of an asthma attack while the patient is sneezing, coughing, or short of breath. The first is responsive pharmaceutical, while the second is prescient pharmaceutical.

4.6. Movement Disorders

In people suffering from Parkinson's disease and movement disorders, the Apple Observe could be used to measure and record dyskinetic symptoms. With Apple Observe, patients can arrange their exercise schedules according to the severity of the indication. Apple Observe Wellbeing helps in analyzing quiet responses to drugs and following the progress of the condition.

4.7. Coagulation Monitoring

A certain number of people's blood coagulation is consistently checked to ensure they remain healthy. When you have a protracted period of blood clotting, you are more likely to experience a stroke or die (for longer than usual). A crisply designed coagulation system allows patients to check their blood clots in real-time via Bluetooth. Rather than going to the clinic frequently, they self-test and transmit discoveries to their health care specialists. Patients may also comment on the results. If the results do not fall within the parameters, the gadget reminds the user to perform the self-test.

4.8. Depression Monitored through an App

The condition of sadness is different from other physiological clutters. In any case, later advancements in the Internet of Things have made it measurable and preventable. A mobile application has been developed to test and evaluate people suffering from extreme depression (MDD). In a later exploratory study, participants used the app to track their disposition and cognition each day. Even though wearable technology has not yet been widely adopted, it has demonstrated its ability to measure the effect of sadness in real-time. In addition, the program provides data to understand and support a more comprehensive discussion of the still-abstract topic of mental illness.

4.9. Smart Contact Lenses

As a small advance has been made in the field of non-invasive smart glasses, they represent a breakthrough within the Internet of Things (IoT). In terms of wearable gadgets that naturally detect changes in eye measurements, the keen contact focal point is one of the few victories. Obtain a warning that if left untreated, this eye degeneration might progress to glaucoma [22]. CE certification and FDA approval have currently been obtained for this innovation for sale and marketing in Europe and the United States. CE certification and FDA approval have also been obtained for Japan.

4.10. Monitoring Medical Adherence

People with hypertension, diabetes, psychosis, and other ailments don't take medicines because of obscurity. Noncompliance with endorsed drugs leads to more readmissions and clinical issues at healing centers. When a wearable piece of jewelry is worn, it can determine whether the individual will ingest the medication. 90% of the time, Bayesian systems are incorrectly categorizing gulping, drinking water, talking water, and spit swallows. Wearable collars can assess adherence to treatment with impressive accuracy and can assist patients in overlooking almost all of their diseases.

4.11. Cancer Treatment

Our current advancements have prevented many people with rehabilitation problems from being detained at home and have reduced the need for them to visit the rehabilitation center regularly. An arbitrary clinical trial was conducted by the American Society for Clinical Oncology, or ASCO, in 357 patients with head and neck cA Bluetooth-enabled weight and blood weight sleeve was used in conjunction with an application to check for side effects. Every day, the indications and treatment responses of patients are improved by this framework. The CYCORE procedure is widely known, and patients who used it had fewer serious cancer-related side effects than patients who saw their standard specialists week after week. Patients and caregivers can recognize and react quickly to new side effects and side effects with CYCORE.

4.12. Posture Correction

A wearable device called Upright Go teaches patients how to correct their posture with biofeedback. A small vibration is delivered when the person using the device slows down. An avatar displaying the client's position can be seen while the client is wearing the gadget. The avatar gets red when the pose closes, showing that the subject has returned to a healthy position. Additionally, the biofeedback vibration encourages a client to make subtle changes to their posture and decreases the risk of future musculoskeletal problems.

4.13. Hearing Aid

People with hearing loss can benefit from computerized auditory devices, which convert sound waves into sophisticated driving forces and provide correct sound replication. An electronic device's voice and other compactors. Modern aids can be programmed to coordinate with the design of hearing loss. iPhone clients, for instance, can enhance sound quality by using the Live Tune feature of Discuss Units. The work makes it possible for people with hearing disabilities to hear the discourse in active situations.

4.14. Sleep Monitoring

Wearable contraptions can measure sleep changes and suggest ways to improve them. One such device is Beddit. Rest time, heart rate, breathing rate, moisture content, and room temperature are all recorded. Using sleep time information and push notifications, the app helps clients achieve their sleep-time objectives based on their rest designs.

4.15. Early Detection of Alzheimer's

50 million people worldwide are affected by Alzheimer's disease. Dementia cannot currently be cured. When considering medications for dementia neuro degenerations, the condition must be evaluated in its early stages, since side effects can appear only recently. Currently, expensive and intrusive treatments such as PET brain imaging and brain liquid testing are available. The goal is to develop a wearable device that can detect early signs of Alzheimer's disease at a low cost.

4.16. Hospital Internal Monitoring

Clinics can benefit greatly from IoT devices. In healing centers, the therapeutic hardware is tagged with sensors that track their whereabouts in real-time. Defibrillators, nebulizers, wheelchairs, oxygen pumps, and other versatile devices may be offered. In addition, a wearable contraption could provide real-time location data for medical experts. With the prevalence of contaminations, IoT-enabled cleanliness devices can actuate whenever health and sanitation conditions require it.

4.17. Respiratory Disease Detection

Sensors that monitor breathing patterns, heart rate, and temperature can alert Smartphone patients to changes in breathing designs, heart rate, and temperature. By monitoring these signals, early deterioration in lung function can be detected. Exacerbations that require immediate attention can be communicated by the app. Near-real-time monitoring of breathing can help assess the condition and prevent it from improving, allowing the therapeutic team to treat it early and prevent aspiratory collapse.

4.18. Artificial Kidneys

In hospitals around the world, hemodialysis is the most common treatment for people with renal failure. A manufactured kidney can improve the lives of patients with renal insufficiency, given the current trends in wearable innovation. Recent Arkansas College research brings us one step closer to prosthetic kidneys. Researchers have developed an engineered nephron that is the same as biological nephrons and can channel blood. Using nanofiltration, ultrafiltration, and turn-around osmosis, this nephron could be coordinated into manufactured kidneys.

4.19. Blood Sensors

The team at Broils Sensor Innovation developed a non-invasive wearable sensor for remote monitoring of key blood components such as glucose, ketones, lactate, urea, and ethanol. Infrared laser spectroscopy is employed by the wearable sensor to distinguish rotationally turning atoms. It is expected to be operational by 2021. Often diabetes patients can test their blood glucose levels without puncturing their fingers without affecting their well-being.

4.20. Lung Monitoring

World Wellbeing Organization data suggests that CHOs are the world's leading cause of death, accounting for a significant number of deaths worldwide. By collecting sound and electrical tomography information at the same time, the WELMO venture intends to build and test low-cost, low-power thermometric sensors that can be integrated into a smart coat and effectively screen the lungs. By assessing lung wellbeing and working precisely and completely in real-time, it will help to assess the adequacy of treatment for persistent obstructive lung diseases.

5. Many Models of Health Care

5.1. IoT in Health Care

The Internet of Things (IoT) could be characterized as a combination of ubiquitous communication, networks, and processing, as well as environmental data. IoT (Internet of Things) is also referred to as IoMT (Web of Therapeutic Things) in health care innovation. In the next decade, there will be 50 billion electronic medical devices. Approximately 847 Zettabytes (ZB) of data will be generated by all IoT devices by 2021, according to Cisco. The Internet of Things will become the world's largest source of information in the long run. Furthermore, it offers health care professionals essential information, such as recognizable evidence, monitoring, and data, allowing issues to be identified early, and fostering improved care administration [3].

5.2. AI in Health Care

By assisting in the elucidation and conclusion of restorative pictures, artificial intelligence in restorative care can improve quiet care and workplace efficiency. Watson, IBM's shrewd cloud, houses one of the most unmistakable AI organizations in health care. Machine learning has effortlessly offered a person considered as a characteristic of intelligent medical solutions for decades. As vital partners within the health care sector profit from and accelerate the care process, the machine learning health care industry takes advantage of and accelerates the care process [24].

5.3. Big Data in Health Care

Health care firms may be able to offer patients more effective strategies and information about their well-being with the help of huge amounts of data. There is a colossal amount of information accessible within the health division, such as budgetary, clinical, R&D, organization, and operational data, which helps to enhance company productivity. By 2019, huge investments in the investment in health care are forecast to reach

5.4. Cloud Computing in Health Care

Cloud computing innovation, which followed huge information, has made health care gear more brilliant. Since cloud computing advances have been taking a toll on investment funds, adaptability, and framework adaptability, the requirement for cloud computing health care services has expanded rapidly with the growing use of cloud-based therapeutic collaboration services.

5.5. Smart Wearables in Health Care

Smart wearables have recently assumed an increasingly significant role in health care and are expected to be a large and promising market in the technology industry, primarily in the form of cardiac diagrams, electroencephalography (EEG), electromyography (EMG), blood pressure (BP), photoplethysmography (PPG), heart-sound, respiration, sleep, and motion surveillance.

5.6. 3D Printing in Health Care

Clinical researchers proposed to use 3D printing to create progressively complex inserts for harrowed patients with the advancement of 3D printing. Furthermore, clinicians want to use 3D printing to create unused hands, feet, legs, noses, and eyes for patients [25]. Clinicians have proposed to use 3D printing to design increasingly complex inserts for beset patients as 3D printing advances. In addition, clinicians should utilize 3D printing to fabricate modern hands, feet, legs, noses, and eyes for patients [25].

6. Key Applications of AI and IoT in Smart Health Care

On the Web, objects could be viewed and accessed in phenomenal ways, a concept known as the Web of Things. Gadgets may collect, analyze, or share information directly or indirectly via an information communication network, while the insights generated by the Web of Things framework are another. Web of Things (IoT) is subsequently a system used in real-life advances, including sensors, arrange associations, counterfeit insights, cloud computing, and vast data. This was done so optimal performance and control could be achieved [26]. Several days have passed since health care providers and device manufacturers integrated AI and IoT in developing sophisticated medicines and devices capable of providing personalized care, beginning with patient diagnosis, hospitals, and the health care sector, while addressing a variety of issues [25].

7. IOT Applications in Health Care

7.1. Real-Time Services Based on Location

Patients' locations can be tracked using IoT. This is especially useful for injured individuals who arrive in a hospital for emergency medical treatment. Real-time monitoring is also made possible with IoT devices, such as room temperature sensors [27].

7.2. Improve Patient Experience

The patient experience is enhanced by IoT devices. The seamless connection between devices allows patients to control the temperature and lighting in their rooms, interact with friends and family, and contact nurses via an intercom. IoT also makes it easier for medical staff to access patient information stored in the cloud [28].

7.3. Hygiene Compliance

The most effective way to prevent infection is to keep your hands clean. Monitoring hand hygiene helps health care professionals determine and establish a level of cleanliness. The most basic function of IoT devices for hand hygiene is to beep when medical personnel approach the bed without washing their hands first.

7.4. Remote Monitoring

IoT is primarily used for remote health monitoring. The treatment that patients receive is adequate when they are monitored continuously. Around the world, many people die from not receiving timely medical care. IoT has the power to address this problem. Complex algorithms and analysis can be applied to IoT devices. Patients in remote locations - where doctors cannot physically travel - can now receive more medical care and attention.

8. Present Applications of AI in Medical Diagnostics

AI may improve patient care and efficacy by assisting with the interpretation and diagnosis of medical images [29].

8.1. Diagnosis and Identification of Diseases

Health care machine learning addresses problems such as illness identification and diagnosis, among others. It combines cognitive computing with genetic tumor sequencing to make precision medicine possible. IBM Watson Genomics is a joint venture with Quest Diagnostics.

8.2. Personalized Treatment/Behavioural Modification

Health data-driven personalized medicine has a strong link to better sickness assessment. The field combines real-time health data with predictive analytics to offer more effective treatment plans. Presently, this sector is governed by supervised learning, which allows doctors to search for genetic information and symptoms within limited diagnoses.

8.3. Drug Development & Discovery

Machine learning has numerous applications in drug research and development, both now and in the future, ranging from next-generation sequencing to precision medicine. In some cases, early drug screening could utilize machine learning algorithms to predict the success rate of treatment based on a range of biological characteristics. MIT and Microsoft are utilizing machine learning algorithms to enhance and better understand diseases and improve therapy.

8.4. Generating Electronic Smart Records

With the increasing amount of data available on medical and health care systems, the development of smart electronic health records, which incorporate artificial intelligence or machine learning, has become increasingly critical for machine-learning applications, which incorporate artificial intelligence or machine learning to maintain health records, interpret health conditions, and propose treatment.

8.5. Automation Machine Learning Systems

Future health care systems might use robotic surgeons as a form of automation. The use of machine learning and deep learning techniques could eventually eliminate the need for human surgeons, allowing robots to operate on patients.

8.6. Radiation Treatments

Early results from artificial intelligence (AI) systems show promise for planning radiotherapy for patients with head and neck cancer.

9. Wearables Technology

Wearable electronics are the next big leap in technology after smartphones.

The term wearable refers to electronic devices or gadgets that can be worn on the body. Using wearable gadgets, real-time data can be collected and analyzed. You can sync your daily activities to your mobile device or laptop using motion sensors. Wearable technology comes in various forms, but activity trackers and smartwatches are among the most popular. Fitbit, Apple Watch, and Samsung Galaxy Gear are just a few examples, as shown in Figure 3.

The internet can be accessed via wearable gadgets and data can be collected in many ways. Users can validate their readings using smartphones and websites. Others allow third parties to view data, such as health care managers or clinicians searching for troubling trends that require medical attention. Often, fitness gadgets encourage users to share their accomplishments on social media with friends and colleagues. A wearable medical device can record any changes to the patient's body immediately [22].

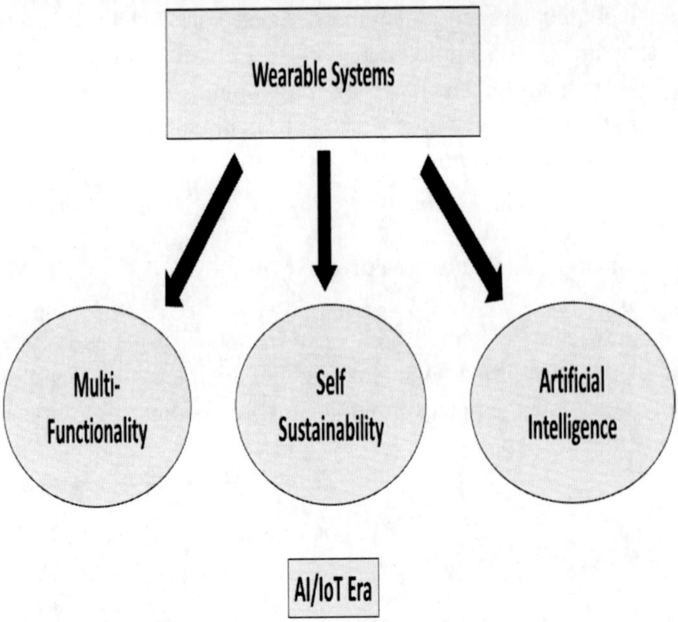

Figure 3. Wearable Systems.

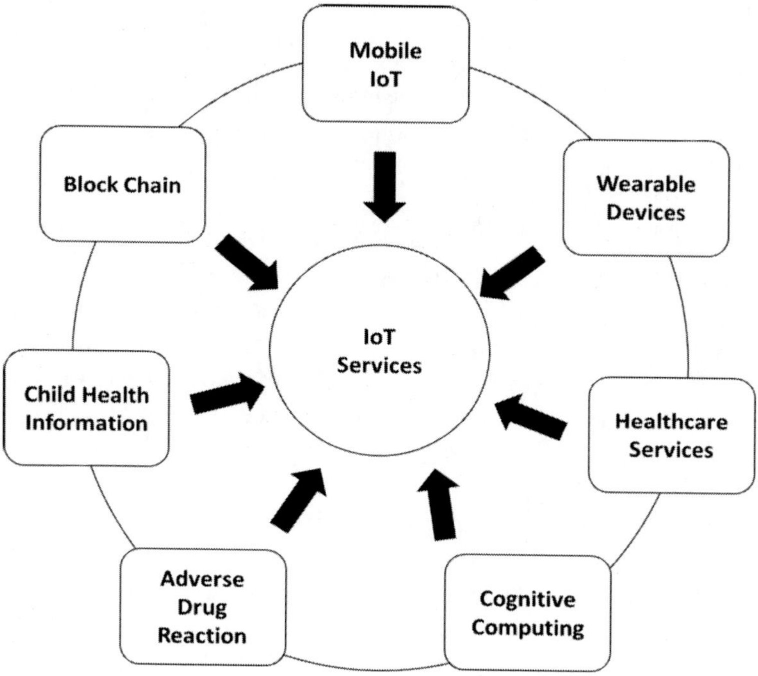

Figure 4. IoT Services to Health care.

Figure 4 depicts an excellent example of someone who suffers from congestive heart failure and recovers at home. By detecting changes in weight, breathing rate, and pulse oxygen level, the device can alert someone when their health is deteriorating. Impact on a variety of industries, but health care has been the primary beneficiary [24]. Through the implementation of wearables, hospitals and clinics can benefit from numerous degrees and responsibilities.

9.1. Encourages Proactive Health Care

Health care can be made more proactive with wearable technology. Wearables may be used to intervene at an early stage as opposed to addressing health concerns afterward. Irregularities Patients who are predisposed to health problems can identify irregularities before they become an issue.

9.2. Keeps Patients Engaged

When they can manage their health using wearable devices, they will be more engaged with it. With the help of a wearable device, users could keep track of their health in real-time.

9.3. Monitors Vulnerable Patients

Health care professionals can also use wearable technology to monitor weak individuals prone to medical problems. It is possible to monitor your loved ones at home if they are in danger, but it is not necessary.

9.4. Improve Patient Care and Satisfaction

To improve decision-making while increasing patient engagement, surgeons and doctors need critical information. One example is to use intelligent lenses to observe patient life and critical information during surgery without removing the patient's eyes.

9.5. Benefits Health Care Providers and Employers

Health care practitioners can gain enormous benefits from wearable technology. The use of wearable devices to screen understanding data can help therapeutic experts better understand issues plaguing patients for a long time. Once you have the data, you can create an analysis that is more precise than you could without the device.

10. IoT and Machine Learning Algorithm

Machine learning involves the use of probability and optimization hypotheses to automate repetitive tasks that cannot be completed procedurally or consistently. By preparing computers for certain information, you could move forward figures or highlights. Admissions vary according to the problem. As part of another program, the data gathered from the apparatus, such as arrangement [29, 30], the same arrangement, or arrangement [29-30], could be incorporated. Amounts of computer control, machine learning models reveal rules that are beyond the capabilities of the human More information is better in a demonstration.

10.1. Artificial Neural Networks

Often, this type of learning approach is called neuronal organizing. Based on the structure and utility of biological brain systems, it is a computational process. By resolving the complicated relationships between inputs and outputs, it is commonly used to identify information designs. Health care forecasts are handled by ANNs, which specialists and specialists cannot manage alone. Cancer and heart problems can be detected by ANNs. Pee and blood tests are analyzed with ANN, diabetics' glucose levels are assessed, particle liquid levels are determined, and different sickness conditions can be distinguished [21].

10.2. Inductive Logic Programming (ILP)

Coherent programming gives this process the power to run input tests, foundation information, and suspicions. A logical reasoning program can be made if any known foundation information is encoded in a consistent real database. This document acknowledges positive opportunities but not negative ones, and it acknowledges speculation in any computer dialect.

10.3. Clustering

Different types of information are relegated to partitioned clusters so that all perceptions within the same cluster are comparable based on already defined standards. By comparing information clusters, similarities between them can be discovered.

10.4. Bayesian Networks

A probabilistic graphical demonstration in which the random variables and their conditions are portrayed using a coordinated, non-cyclic diagram. One could, for instance, present the probabilistic relationship between different ailments and their side effects. By knowing the warning signs, we can assess the risk of different illnesses in this organization.

10.5. Decision Tree Learning

The choice tree approach is a machine learning approach that employs a choice tree to demonstrate an expectation. In this way, perceptions about an object are linked with different suspicions about its objective value. In a health care setting, a choice tree analysis is often used when treatment choices or results are unclear, and such choices and results are important (wellbeing, affliction, or death). As a result, specialists are in a better position to select the best treatment option for their patients.

Conclusion

Health care has benefited greatly from the Internet of Things. Health care delivery costs and the frequency of doctor and hospital visits are significantly lowered by the Internet of Things. Sensors are also useful for collecting data that can be utilized to help prevent disease progression. As a result, they can rethink their goods, services, and development. To manage their health, patients are embracing medical IoT devices. Manufacturers of medical devices try to offer more accurate, intelligent, and personalized solutions. Wearable technology also has a bright future in the digital health care sector, from the perspective of a patient. In addition, it highlights how this could lead to more efficient and cost-effective health care delivery.

References

Ahad, M. Tahir, and K.-L. A. Yau, "5G-based smart Health care network: architecture, taxonomy, challenges and future research directions," *IEEE Access*, vol. 7, pp. 100747–100762, 2019.

B. Oryema, "Design and implementation of an interoperable messaging system for IoT Health care services," in *Proceedings of the 2017 14th IEEE Annual Consumer Communications & Networking Conference (CCNC)*, pp. 45–52, Las Vegas, NV, USA, January 2017.

C. Tsirmpas, A. Anastasiou, P. Bountris, and D. Koutsouris, "A new method for profile generation in an internet of things environment: an application in ambient-assisted living," *IEEE Internet of Things Journal*, vol. 2, no. 6, pp. 471–478, 2015.

D. P. Young, "Ultra-wideband (UWB) transmitter location using time difference of arrival (TDOA) techniques," in *Proceedings of The Thirty-Seventh Asilomar Conference on Signals, Systems & Computers*, pp. 1225–1229, Pacific Grove, CA, USA, November 2003.

Dohr, "The internet of things for ambient assisted living," in *Proceedings of the 2010 Seventh International Conference on Information Technology: New Generations*, pp. 804–809, Las Vegas, NA, USA, April 2010.

E. Qin, "Cloud computing and the internet of things: technology innovation in automobile service," in *Proceedings of the International Conference on Human Interface and the Management of Information*, pp. 173–180, Las Vegas, NV, USA, July 2013.

Froiz-Míguez, T. Fernández-Caramés, P. Fraga-Lamas, and L. Castedo, "Design, implementation and practical evaluation of an IoT home automation system for fog computing applications based on MQTT and ZigBee-WiFi sensor nodes," *Sensors*, vol. 18, no. 8, p. 2660, 2018.

G. Cerruela García, I. Luque Ruiz, and M. Gómez-Nieto, "State of the art, trends, and future of Bluetooth low energy, near field communication and visible light communication in the development of smart cities," *Sensors*, vol. 16, no. 11, p. 1968, 2016.

G. Marques and R. Pitarma, "An indoor monitoring system for ambient assisted living based on internet of things architecture," *International Journal of Environmental Research and Public Health*, vol. 13, no. 11, p. 1152, 2016.

G. Shanmugasundaram and G. Sankarikaarguzhali, "An investigation on IoT Health care analytics," *International Journal of Information Engineering and Electronic Business*, vol. 9, no. 2, p. 11, 2017.

G. Yang, L. Xie, M. Mantysalo, et al., "A health-IoT platform based on the integration of intelligent packaging, unobtrusive bio-sensor, and intelligent medicine box," *IEEE Transactions on Industrial Informatics*, vol. 10, no. 4, pp. 2180–2191, 2014.

Gatouillat, Y. Badr, B. Massot, and E. Sejdic, "Internet of medical things: a review of recent contributions dealing with cyber-physical systems in medicine," *IEEE Internet of Things Journal*, vol. 5, no. 5, pp. 3810–3822, 2018.

H. Aftab, K. Gilani, J. Lee, L. Nkenyereye, S. Jeong, and J. Song, "Analysis of identifiers in IoT platforms," *Digital Communications and Networks*, vol. 6, no. 3, pp. 333–340, 2020.

H. Peng, Y. Tian, J. Kurths, L. Li, Y. Yang, and D. Wang, "Secure and energy-efficient data transmission system based on chaotic compressive sensing in body-to-body networks," *IEEE Transactions on Biomedical Circuits and Systems*, vol. 11, no. 3, pp. 558–573, 2017.

J.-Y. Lee and R. A. Scholtz, "Ranging in a dense multipath environment using a UWB radio link," *IEEE Journal on Selected Areas in Communications*, vol. 20, pp. 1677–1683, 2002.

K. T. Kadhim, "An overview of patient's health status monitoring system based on internet of things (IoT)," *Wireless Personal Communications*, vol. 114, pp. 1–28, 2020.

L. M. Dang, M. J. Piran, D. Han, K. Min, and H. Moon, "A survey on internet of things and cloud computing for Health care," *Electronics*, vol. 8, no. 7, p. 768, 2019.

L. Syed, S. Jabeen, M. S., and A. Alsaeedi, "Smart Health care framework for ambient assisted living using IoT and big data analytics techniques," *Future Generation Computer Systems*, vol. 101, pp. 136–151, 2019.

M. Khan, K. Han, and S. Karthik, "Designing smart control systems based on internet of things and big data analytics," *Wireless Personal Communications*, vol. 99, no. 4, pp. 1683–1697, 2018.

M. N. Birje and S. S. Hanji, "Internet of things based distributed Health care systems: a review," Journal of Data, Information, and Management, vol. 2, 2020.

P. J. Nachankar, "IoT in agriculture," Decision Making, vol. 1, no. 3, 2018.

P. S. Mathew, "Applications of IoT in Health care," in *Cognitive Computing for Big Data Systems over IoT*, pp. 263–288, Springer, Berlin, Germany, 2018.

R. J. Fontana and S. J. Gunderson, "Ultra-wideband precision asset location system," in *Proceedings of the 2002 IEEE Conference on Ultra-Wideband Systems and Technologies (IEEE Cat. No. 02EX580)*, pp. 147–150, Baltimore, MD, USA, May 2002.

R. Peng and M. L. Sichitiu, "Angle of arrival localization for wireless sensor networks," in *Proceedings of the 2006 3rd Annual IEEE Communications Society on Sensor and Ad Hoc Communications and Networks*, pp. 374–382, Reston, Virginia, September 2006.

R. Zetik, "UWB localization-active and passive approach [ultra wideband radar]," in *Proceedings of the 21st IEEE Instrumentation and Measurement Technology Conference (IEEE Cat. No. 04CH37510)*, pp. 1005–1009, Como, Italy, May 2004.

V. G. Menon, *"An IoT-enabled intelligent automobile system for smart cities," Internet of Things*, p. 100213, 2020.

V. Jagadeeswari, "A study on medical Internet of Things and Big Data in the personalized Health care system," *Health Information Science And Systems*, vol. 6, p. 14, 2018.

Y. Yan, "A home-based health information acquisition system," *Health Information Science and Systems*, vol. 1, p. 12, 2013.

Y. Yuehong, "The internet of things in Health care: an overview," *Journal of Industrial Information Integration*, vol. 1, pp. 3–13, 2016.

Z. Ali, M. S. Hossain, G. Muhammad, and A. K. Sangaiah, "An intelligent Health care system for detection and classification to discriminate vocal fold disorders," *Future Generation Computer Systems*, vol. 85, pp. 19–28, 2018.

Chapter 6

Polycystic Ovarian Syndrome at a High Rise in Jammu and Kashmir - Its Early Prediction Using Decision Tree Classification Techniques

Anjume Shakir*
M. tech (CSE) Scholar, Desh Bhagat University, Mandi Gobindgarh, Pujab, India

Abstract

Polycystic Ovarian syndrome (PCOS) is the complex ovarian ailment that affects the healthy life of women. The excessive formation of follicular cysts in the ovaries is the cause of this problem which in turn leads to infertility and even cancer in later stages. It is characterized by counting the number of follicles in ovary. This disorder is at high rise in Jammu and Kashmir from last few decades. The study shows that about 29% of the teenage girls are suffering from this disorder. The disorder is incurable but treatable if diagnosed at the early age. In this paper the utilization of machine learning techniques for early prediction of Polycystic Ovarian Syndrome will be presented. Since the actual causes for the PCOS are yet not known and the disorder is incurable but treatable. The Early diagnosis of PCOS can help patients to take the necessary precautions and treatment required to fight it. The paper presents the implementation of Decision Tree Classification to predict the PCOS at early stage.

Keywords: PCOS, stress, machine learning, hormonal imbalance, early prediction

---

*Corresponding Author's Email: ashakir01@gmail.com.

In: AI-Enabled IoT for Smart Health Care Systems
Editors: Tawseef Ayoub Shaikh, Tabasum Rasool and Mohammed Wasid
ISBN: 978-1-68507-977-2

1. Introduction

Polycystic Ovary Syndrome (PCOS), a hormonal imbalance mostly found in mature women. PCOS affects 6 to 10% of women globally and half of them go undiagnosed. In India 10-15% of the women are affected by this disorder. PCOS is engulfing Jammu and Kashmir also with high pace. The Indian Council of Medical Research (ICMR) reports that 29% of the teenage girls in Jammu and Kashmir show early signs of PCOS [1]. The findings show that 52% of the patients diagnosed of PCOS are suffering from high rates of stress and anxiety disorders like Generalized Anxiety Disorder (GAD). It hints of the close relation between PCOS and stress [2]. Patients suffering from menstrual irregularities develop the hormonal imbalance which leads to the infertility, diabetes and other diseases at later stages. Since the actual reason for the PCOS are unknown till date but the researchers believe that food habits, obesity, stress and less physical activity are believed to be the reasons for developing this disorder [3].

PCOS, discovered by Stein and Leventhal in the year 1935, sometimes also branded as Stein-Leventhal Syndrome. PCOS is the hormonal imbalance balance characterized by hyperandrogenism, in which excess quantity of androgens, Estrogens, Progesterone, Luteinizing hormones are secreted which leads to hirsutism and amenorrhea[4]. These excessive hormones develop the follicles in ovaries which later on become cysts and hinder normal menstruation and ovulation and become the reason for the infertility in future.

Data mining has application in predicting some diseases like cancer, diabetes, heart disease etc at the early stage and the proper treatments can be done after the analysis of the results. In some of the diseases like heart disease, the accuracy achieved good. Applying, data mining for the early prediction and possible fertility chances can prove very fruitful for the doctors and patients as well. In Data mining the dataset of the PCOS patients taken from the authentic sources, analyzed and then the particular machine learning algorithms are applied to predict the results. It not only saves their money of the patients but also assists them in getting the results quick and accurate.

2. Literature Review

Since much work has not been done over the prediction of PCOS using the data mining but some efforts have been made by researchers. The PCOS is believed to be caused do to obesity and less physical activity but the actual causes are yet to be discovered. Ranjitha Sitheswaran et al., [5], did literature inspection of the Polycystic Ovarian Morphology (PCOM) and presented the causes, symptoms and associated diseases with PCOS. M. Alotaibi, A. Alsinan [6], in their case study on PCOS on Gulf Countries and presented the system supported by mobile health care technologies using statistical software. Sandy Rihana et al., [7], proposed an automated cysts detection and classification of ovary using multi-scale morphology and SVM. Sharvari S. et al., [8], proposed an automated detection of PCOS by calculating no of follicles from ultrasound report and along with the assimilation of other clinical factors to classify patients in PCOS and Normal. Yinhui Deng et al., [9], introduced adaptive morphological filter and watershed algorithm to extract outlines of targets, a clustering to identify to expected follicular cysts. Palak Mehrotra et al., [10], published a paper in Automated Ovarian Follicle Recognition for Polycystic Ovary Syndrome used the techniques like multi-scale morphological approach for contrast Enhancement and scanline thresholding is used to extract the contours of the follicles. Neetha Thomas et al., [11], did survey on causes, symptoms, treatments and associated diseases of the women suffering from PCOS. Vikas B et al., [12] studied different applications of data mining techniques in the field of medicine that can be extended for further research of PCOS.

3. Symptoms and Treatment

PCOS develops from the small age therefore takes time to find the symptoms related to this disorder. Just from ultrasound report one cannot make diagnosis of PCOS, Body Mass Index (BMI), menstrual cycles and by identifying of the other symptoms can help in correct diagnosis.

The major PCOS symptoms are:

a. Hirsutism (growing of body hairs, acne and male like baldness) [13] [14, 15]
b. Irregularities in menstruation cycles [16, 17]
c. Abnormalities in ovulation. d. Hormonal imbalance [18]
d. Weight gain, headache and Risk of depression [19]
e. Cardio vascular disorders [20]
f. Excess number of follicles in ovary [17].

This problem mainly takes place due to over secretion of the male hormones (hyperandrogenism). Thus the disorder is recognized by the generation of characteristics in females like male like baldness, growing of excessive body hairs, acne, rough skin patches in places like calves, armpits etc. and dark skin tone. All these symptoms fall in Hirsutism.

Hormonal imbalance even affects normal monthly cycle because of the delay in the ovulation. Doctors believe that if the patient's cycle length is constantly more than 32 days, may be sign of the PCOS. The other symptoms related to this also include the excessive bleeding and constant pain during the cycles. Body Mass index (BMI) is measured by weight per meter square. Obesity is one of the main reasons which can lead to PCOS. Doctors periodically check the weight of the patients to make sure that it does not cross 24 kg/m^2 because as per World Health Organization (WHO), people with BMI above 24 kg/m^2 are considered to be overweight.

In Jammu and Kashmir one of the main reasons for PCOS is "Stress," due to the prevalent situation of the state for last few decades. Since stress consists of sub factors like high blood pressure, fatigue, depression, insomnia, headache, digestive problems, sleeplessness etc. When the most of sub symptoms are identified in the patient by doctor, the patient is said to be suffering from stress. Treatment includes developing a healthy lifestyle and maintaining the proper diet. Weight loss and regular exercise are proving to be very effective for PCOS. Oral contraceptives also help in regulating the menstrual cycles and help in ovulation. Since the disorder has genetic as well as environmental causes therefore for Jammu and Kashmir, the depression and stress are considered to be the one of the cause of the PCOS. In such case stress free environment can be one of the fruitful solutions to counter the disorder.

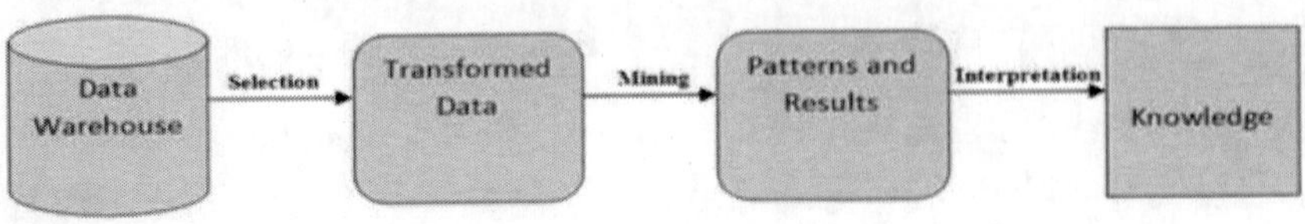

Figure 1. Data mining process.

4. Datamining Techniques

Data mining is the branch of computer science that deals with the finding of patters in large data, involving methods of machine learning, artificial intelligence and database systems. Data mining implies use of software and intelligence on the dataset to infer new information. Figure 1 depicts the data mining process and the techniques involved in retrieving the information.

Data mining techniques mainly include Classification, Regression, Clustering and Association which are used as per the requirement for classification, prediction, visualization, deviation detection and pattern finding. Data mining has application in business, marketing, Artificial Intelligence, user behavior, health and science. In the field of health care, lot of valuable work has been incorporated on diagnosis of some chronic diseases in preliminary stage like prediction of cancer [21], diabetes [22], etc.

5. Approach

Only the follicle count from the ultrasound report is not enough for the diagnosis of this disorder [23]. Therefore other factors are taken into consideration in predicting the PCOS accurately. The factors that have been selected for obtaining the results are tabulated in Table 1.

Lot of factors were identified which are responsible for the PCOS. The preprocessing of the attributes was done using the filter and wrapper techniques which are independent of data mining techniques. The attributes which contribute majorly in causing the disorder where filtered and the best subset of attributes where selected.

Table 1. Factors to predict PCOS

Factors	Normal Values	Attribute Values
No. of Follicles	>10	[<10, 10-20, >20]
BMI (kg/m^2)	>24	[YES, NO]
Cycle Length (days)	>32	[YES, NO]
FSH (IU/L)	>5	[<5, 5-8, >8]
Stress	Present/Absent	[YES, NO]

```
=== Detailed Accuracy By Class ===

                 TP Rate  FP Rate  Precision  Recall   F-Measure  MCC      ROC Area  PRC Area  Class
                 0.889    0.091    0.889      0.889    0.889      0.798    0.818     0.797     NORMAL
                 0.909    0.111    0.909      0.909    0.909      0.798    0.818     0.826     PCOS
Weighted Avg.    0.900    0.102    0.900      0.900    0.900      0.798    0.818     0.813

=== Confusion Matrix ===

  a  b   <-- classified as
  8  1 |  a = NORMAL
  1 10 |  b = PCOS
```

Figure 2. Accuracy and Confusion matrix (Weka).

Patient	Follicles	FSH	Cycle mon	BMI	Stress	Diagnosis
A105	10 to 20	5 to 8	NO	YES	NO	NORMAL
A106	10 to 20	5 to 8	NO	NO	YES	NORMAL
A108	10 to 20	<5	YES	YES	NO	PCOS
A109	10 to 20	<5	YES	NO	YES	PCOS
A110	10 to 20	<5	NO	YES	NO	NORMAL
A112	<10	>8	YES	YES	NO	PCOS
A113	<10	>8	YES	NO	YES	PCOS
A114	<10	>8	NO	NO	YES	NORMAL
A115	<10	5 to 8	YES	YES	YES	PCOS
A117	<10	5 to 8	NO	NO	NO	NORMAL
A120	<10	<5	YES	YES	YES	NORMAL

Figure 3. Data set.

Taking these factors into consideration algorithm we can use classification techniques of machine learning and divide the patients into two class PCOS and Normal patients. The supervised machine learning technique will be used trained used a part of the dataset and the remaining dataset will be used as the test data. As per the study 39% of the patients have elevated hormones levels like Testosterone, LH and FSH.59% of the patients are diagnosed with obesity and 15% with non-timely menstrual cycle. As per the findings 52% of patients in Kashmir suffering from some stress are diagnosed with PCOS [2]. The Dataset was prepared after getting the manual data from the gynecologists working in the field. The dataset was preprocessed before classification is applied on it, Figure 3 depicts the dataset considered.

With all the things on board we found that based on these factors, PCOS could be predicted early. The classification technique we have used to classify the Normal and PCOS patients is Decision tree, a supervised machine learning technique. Decision tree is covering both classification and regression in a way and help in making the classification tree. The decision analysis is used explicitly in making the correct and quick decisions. The reason behind using Decision Tree is its simplicity and clear visualization, interpretation, implicit feature selection and can handle numerical as well as categorical data. J48 classifier is an extension of ID3 (Iterative Dichotomiser 3) and accounts for decision trees pruning, missing values, ranges of continuous attribute values, rule derivation, etc. Since WEKA tool bestows with numerous options associated with the tree pruning. The WEKA tool was used to get the results by taking the required data. The dataset structure and results of the WEKA tool are given in Figure 2 and Figure 3 respectively.

Conclusion

Using the Decision Tree classification technique, the results show 90% precision and the use of machine learning techniques will help in predicting the PCOS easily by taking some related factors in consideration. The results achieved will obviously be faster and accurate than the manual doctor visits. In this paper lot of symptoms of PCOS have been enumerated lot but after feature extraction we were able to find some important factors responsible for PCOS viz; follicles, BMI, cycle length, quantity of hormones (LH and FSH) and stress. The accuracy of prediction depends on the size of the data set. The Decision Tree classification technique has shown good results for the dataset.

Future Scope

In future large dataset can be taken and different machine learning algorithms are applied to achieve the accuracy of the prediction. The early detection of

PCOS can help the doctors in treating the early stage patients and avoiding the serious issues that will lead due to it. There is scope for predicting the possibilities of conceiving in the PCOS patients using the Machine learning techniques as well.

Acknowledgments

We would like to thank Dr. Shagufta Akther, Gynecologist, Department of Health Services, Government of Jammu and Kashmir for her kind support in explaining the clinical aspects of PCOS and providing the data required for the research.

References

Alotaibi M., A. Alsinan. "Mobile Polycystic Ovarian Syndrome Management and Awareness System for Gulf Countries," *SAI Computing Conference, IEEE*, July 2016.

Balpande V. R. and Rakhi D. Wajgi, "Prediction and severity estimation of diabetes using data mining technique," *International conference on Innovative Mechanisms for Industry Applications*, July 2017.

Cheng J. J. et al., "Data mining and classification of polycystic ovaries in pelvic ultrasound reports," *bioRXiv*, Jan 2018.

Deng Y. et al., "Automated Detection of Polycystic Ovary Syndrome from Ultrasound Images," in *IEEE- 30th Annual International,* British Columbia, Aug 2008.

Doia S. A. R. et al., "Steroidogenic alterations and adrenal androgen excess in PCOS," *Steriods*, Vol. 71, Issue 9, pp. 751-759, Sept 2006.

Luef G., I. Abraham et al., "Hyperandrogenism, postprandial hyperinsulinism and the risk of PCOS in a cross sectional study of women with epilepsy treated with valproate," *Elsevier*, Vol. 48, Issue 1-2, pp. 91-102, Jan 2002.

McAllister J. M. et al., "Functional genomics of PCOS: from GWAS to molecularmechanisms," *Elsevier*, Vol. 26, Issue 3, pp. 118-124, Mar 2015.

Mehrotra P. et al., "Automated Ovarian Follicle Recognition for Polycystic Ovary Syndrome" *IEEE- International Conference on Image Information Processing,* Nov 2011.

Mumtaz R., "Polycystic Ovary Syndrome (PCOS): The 'Silent Disorder' in Kashmiri Women," *Kashmir Life*, Mar 2016.

Polycystic ovary syndrome, http://en.wikipedia.org/wiki/Polycystic_ovary_syndrome.

Ramachandran P. et al., "Early Detection and Prevention of Cancer using Data Mining Techniques," *International Journal of Computer Applications*, Vol. 97, Issue 13, pp. 48-53, July 2014.

Rasool S. Dr., "Polycystic ovary Syndrome," *Greater Kashmir*, pp. 07, Jan 2018.

Rihana S. et al., "Automated Algorithm for Ovarian Cysts Detection in Ultrasonogram," *IEEE 2nd International Conference on Advances in Biomedical Engineering*, Sept 2013.

Roe A. H. et al., "Using the Androgen Excess-PCOS Society Criteria to Diagnose Polycystic Ovary Syndrome and the Risk of Metabolic Syndrome in Adolescents," *The Journal of Pediatrics*, Vol. 162, No. 5, May 2013.

Sahingöz M. et al., "Axis I and Axis II diagnoses in women with PCOS," *Elsevier*, Vol. 35, Issue 5, pp. 508-511, Sept 2013.

Shah S., "Infertility-causing ovarian disorder on rise in Kashmir," *Kashmir Moniter*, Dec 2016.

Sharvari S. et al., "Automated Detection of Polycystic Ovarian Syndrome Using Follicle Recognition," *IEEE International Conference-* (ICACCCT), May 2014.

Sitheswaran R., S. Malarkhodi "An Effective Automated System in Follicle Identification for Polycystic Ovary Syndrome Using Ultrasound Images," *IEEE*, Sept 2014.

Swanton A. et al., "IVF outcome in women with PCOS, PCO and normal ovarian morphology," *European Journal of Obstetrics & Gynecology and Reproductive Biology*, Vol. 149, pp. 68-71, Dec 2010.

Thomas N. and Dr. A. Kavitha, "A Literature Inspection on Polycystic Ovarian Morphology in Women Using Data Mining Methodologies," *International Journal of Advanced Research in Computer Science*, Vol. 9, issue 1, pp. 547-551, Feb 2018.

Vikas B., Sipra Sarangi, Manaswini Chilla, K. Santosh Bhargav and B S Anuhya, "A Literature Review on the Rising Phenomenon PCOS," *International Journal of Advances in Engineering & Technology*, Vol. 10, Issue 2, pp. 216-224, Apr 2017.

Wissing M. L. et al., "Impact of PCOS on early embryo cleavage kinetics," *Reproductive biomedicine online*, Vol. 28, pp. 508-514, Jan 2013.

Chapter 7

Data-Driven Modern Health Care Systems with the Internet of Medical Things Combined with Big Data and Machine Learning

E. Fantin Irudaya Raj*

Department of Electrical and Electronics Engineering, Dr. Sivanthi Aditanar College of Engineering, Tamilnadu, India

Abstract

As the world population expands and the adverse effects of global warming and environmental pollution aggravate, health-related issues are ramping exponentially. Nowadays, health problems are prevalent not only among the elderly but also among those between the ages of 20 to 40. Finding time for a hospital visit and having routine health check-ups is extremely difficult in today's busy world. As a result, there is a need to prioritize remote health monitoring for both patients and physicians. The recent advancements in wireless communications, embedded systems, the Internet of Things (IoT), sensors, and nanotechnology make it possible to monitor the individual's health continuously and remotely. It is possible by wearable or implantable sensory devices, which collects the information of vital health parameters of the individual who wears or implants it. These devices can generate distress signals through a buzzer or alert message when the parameter being monitored crosses a set threshold value. In real-time applications, these devices and the entire health care systems generate a huge volume of data. Traditional data management techniques are often unable to manage these voluminous data. Big Data analytics are overcoming the limitations of traditional data

*Corresponding Author's Email: fantinraj@gmail.com.

In: AI-Enabled IoT for Smart Health Care Systems
Editors: Tawseef Ayoub Shaikh, Tabasum Rasool and Mohammed Wasid
ISBN: 978-1-68507-977-2

management methodologies and bringing a revolution in modern health care systems. In addition to that, Machine Learning (ML) Techniques and their algorithms are effectively managed and trained with this data. It will make the computers predict the health care issues well in advance and make the individuals or doctors take precautionary steps. The present work discusses various wearable or implantable sensory devices used by individuals and the network architecture. And it also discusses the basics and underlying principles of the Internet of Medical Things (IoMT), Big Data, and ML techniques used in data-driven modern health care systems in detail.

Keywords: modern health care system, big data, sensory devices, machine learning, internet of medical things (IoMT), wearable/implantable devices

1. Introduction

Technological advancements have changed the face of modern health care. Modern health care is impacted by the growth of a consumerization culture in which consumers can shop around from relevant providers. In order to remain profitable, medical practice managers must adapt to these conditions by devising approaches that allow them to give unsurpassed patient care (Gope et al., 2020). For the past few years, technology has been utilized in health care to operate specialist equipment such as X-ray machines and magnetic resonance imaging scanners. Increasingly, technology is being employed to enhance the management of more efficient practice and the patient experience (Datta et al., 2020). Along with providing required standards of care, modern health care necessitates adopting new ways of working and communicating with patients.

Medical error is the third greatest cause of death in the United States, behind cancer and heart disease. According to some estimates, the United States loses 4,000 people each year due to medical mistakes. India has a considerably higher death toll. The most common errors are related to diagnosis, prescription, and improper use of medicine. According to the World Health Organization, inadequate health care causes millions of patients to harm each year, resulting in 2.6 million fatalities in underdeveloped and developing nations alone. This epidemic has brought to light the serious flaws in the health care system and the urgent need for technology to address some of those flaws (Stawicki et al., 2019).

In the Western world, practically every country has the same problem: an ageing population that is rapidly increasing. People live longer, and those with noncommunicable diseases (such as diabetes) require continuous medical care and monitoring. Suppose health care is to stay up with this level of demand. In that case, it will need to incorporate today's sophisticated breakthroughs, such as Artificial Intelligence (AI), Data Mining, Deep Learning (DL), Machine Learning (ML), Internet of Medical Things (IoMT), etc. The good news is that AI has already been implemented in the health care industry, though it still needs more widespread adoption to become relatively common. For example, one existing AI program allows scientists to explore and evaluate cancer patients' DNA data. The researchers can utilize AI to discover specific mutations that can categorize the level of danger in patients. This pattern recognition allows for improved screening and overall illness management efficiency (Ahmad et al., 2018).

Doctors are highly trained experts who are sometimes unable to diagnose patients correctly. In such circumstances, AI can assist in making better decisions by quickly handling (assessment and characterization) unwell patients, perhaps saving lives. Decision support systems sift and understand a significant amount of data available within electronic medical records using AI algorithms. In addition, in conjunction with imaging technology, it aids in detecting doubt by identifying issue regions, hence improving the diagnosing process. Finally, AI enhances the relationship between health care providers and patients. In collaboration with physicians and researchers, Artificial intelligence-powered intelligent agents may present, identify, search for, and apply the most up-to-date clinical knowledge, significantly improving clinical efficiency and quality of care (Yu et al., 2018). The research, diagnosis, and analysis of patient data are all part of a doctor's day-to-day responsibilities. Traditionally, a radiologist would look over hundreds of photos to find the greatest match for an X-ray before interpreting it. AI can now automatically determine the best match, as well as some slightly differing ones.

The current work gives insight into the different wearable or implantable sensory devices that people utilize to monitor vital health signs in the modern world. It also explores the fundamentals and underlying ideas of the Big Data, Machine Learning (ML), and Internet of Medical Things (IoMT) approaches employed in today's data-driven health care systems.

2. Modern Health Care System

To meet the new problems and grab new opportunities, modern health care practice can use some common aspects of modern health care. They are a. Wearable tracking and monitoring devices, b. Internet of Medical Things (IoMT), c. Efficient monitoring and recording of information in real-time, d. Modernized doctor-patient communication.

2.1. Wearable Tracking and Monitoring Devices

According to reports, about a 1/4th of Americans owns a wearable gadgets or device for health monitoring. Sleep, fitness, and heart rates can all be tracked with these devices. Consumers are taking an active role in their well-being by connecting wearable devices through their cellphones to monitor and preserve data in this practice of modern health care (Khan et al., 2016). While wearable technology is gaining popularity, some experts believe that adoption may accelerate if doctors can use the data collected by the device to improve patient care. Figure 1 shows a simple wearable device that monitors the person's health data who wears it.

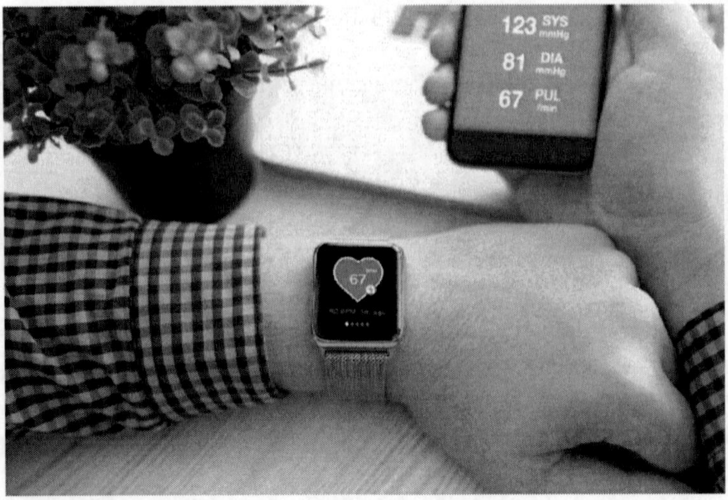

Figure 1. Simple wearable device that monitors health data.

Wearable gadgets have the potential to improve patient health significantly. However, the entire extent to which wearable technologies will affect modern health care is unknown. Numerous studies are presently underway to examine the extent to which wearables can aid in the promotion of a healthy lifestyle. For example, The Universal Research Solutions will collaborate with the Orthopaedic Institute at Geisinger Health System to conduct research using real-time patient data collection. The main goal of this research is to see how data from wearable technology might assist medical practitioners in making better judgments (Hung et al., 2004).

This advanced technology is presently being developed with the goal of improving patient care. "Philips," for example, has developed a wearable medical biosensor that inspects patients as they navigate across the medical center. Among other things, the device will monitor the patient's rate of respiration, body temperature, and pulse rate. Furthermore, the biosensor will be linked to software that will alert the competent caretaker when difficulties arise, allowing them to respond appropriately. Figure 2 illustrates the conventional wireless body area network architecture (WBAN) and numerous implantable and wearable technologies.

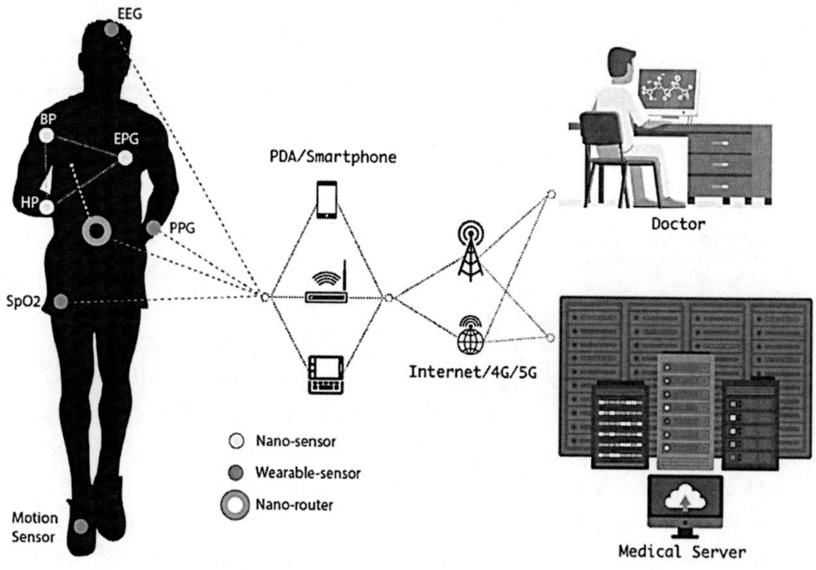

Figure 2. Architecture of a Conventional Wireless Body Area Network (WBAN).

WBAN is made up of several components and has a distinct architecture. The structure can be broken down into various segments. The first section consists of the sensor node, nano-sensor node, and sensory devices implanted within or on the person's body. These economical devices are equipped with physiological and movement sensors that are individually placed on various body parts to monitor specific activities. The sensors can connect wirelessly with the base station directly or via nano-routers strategically positioned across the network to maintain a consistent data flow. Additionally, it results in a reduction in sensor power consumption when transmitting data to the base station, which is especially beneficial for in-body sensors. The second section is the base station or gateway, which is responsible for connecting all nodes in the network. The gateway can be a nearby Wi-Fi router or a mobile phone that communicates with the control unit via the internet or a cellular network (Khan et al., 2012).

This gateway has a higher energy and processing capacity, which enables it to undertake some preliminary analysis, such as submitting a request to collect data from a specific sensor, analyzing the received data, or performing an initial assessment of the monitored activity's state. The cloud system is the final section. It could be medical equipment or a computer used by a physician to assess a patient's health, or it could be an emergency service dispatching medical assistance in an emergency. More research on how wearable technologies might help modern health care is needed. Encourage movement and exercise with wearable technology, on the other hand, is a straightforward way for the patient to employ this technology to improve their health care monitoring.

2.2. Internet of Medical Things (IoMT)

The IoMT is a collection of medical equipment and applications that can communicate with health care information technology systems via networking technologies. By linking patients to their physicians and allowing for the secure transmission of medical data, it is possible to eliminate unnecessary hospital visits and the strain on health care systems. The IoMT market is comprised of smart devices such as wearables and medical/vital monitors used only for health care purposes on the body, in the home, or in community, clinic, or hospital settings, as well as associated real-time location, telehealth, and other services (Pustokhina et al., 2020). Figure 3 depicts the IoMT and its various applications and implementations.

The rise of the Internet of Medical Things (IoMT) accelerated the emergence of implantable and wearable devices, delivering on the anticipation of more affordable treatment and disease management. In contemporary health care, the IoMT has a broad array of applications. Medical device integration and remote monitoring are two examples. The goal of bringing the Internet of Things (IoT) into mainstream health care seems to be to increase patient engagement and allow physicians to the management of chronic conditions (Qureshi et al., 2018). The Internet of Medical Things has a variety of effects on the health care industry. The most visible improvements occur when it is utilized in hospitals, the community, on the body, and at home.

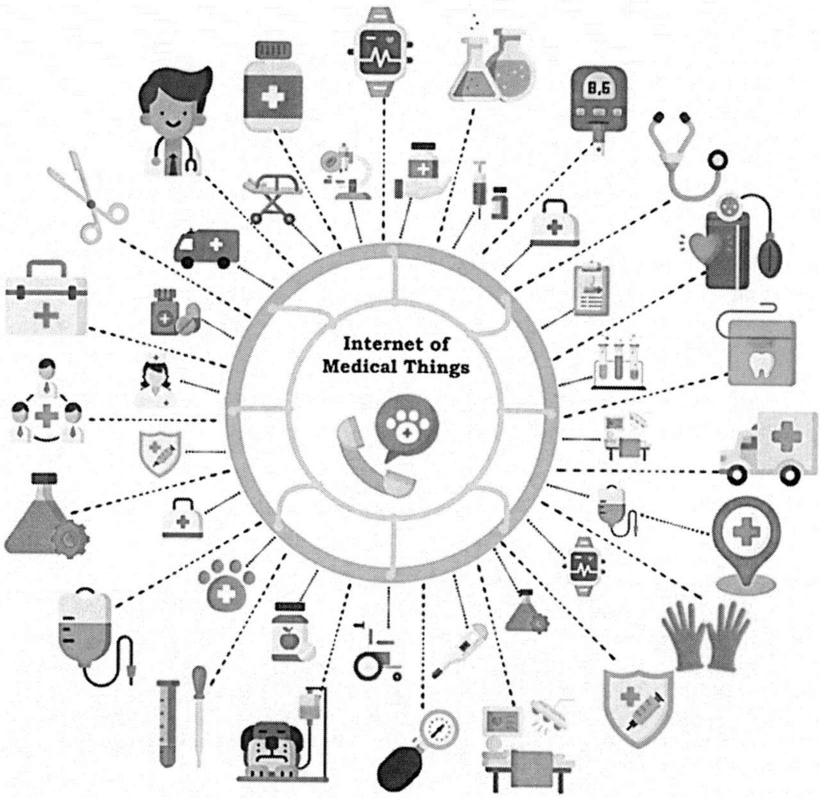

Figure 3. IoMT and its Various Applications.

2.2.1. IoMT Used in Home

Individuals can utilise in-home IoMT to send health records from their homes to other locations, such as a hospital or a primary care clinic. The procedure of sending metrics like oxygen saturation and blood pressure from recently discharged patients to their hospitals for review by their doctors is known as remote patient monitoring (RPM). It can help prevent rehospitalizations to the hospital by identifying problems early on. Telehealth is a term that refers to the use of communication technologies to provide remote health care services. It adds to the flexibility by allowing newly discharged patients to communicate with their doctors remotely to handle small difficulties. Outside of the patient context, IoMT devices in conjunction with telehealth can be beneficial for ongoing treatment. Personal emergency response systems (PERS), for example, can detect and automatically summon help in the event of a heart attack or a fall. Additionally, PERS might provide safeguard for vulnerable individuals, like elders who desire to live independently but are concerned about their safety.

2.2.2. On-Body IoMT

Wearable medical equipment that is linked to remote monitoring systems are referred to on-body IoMT. It is portable and may be utilized outside the home while individuals go about their regular routines. These devices are wearable health monitors that anybody can purchase for personal use or to share with health care providers. It can also provide early warning indicators for more serious health concerns, in addition to measuring basic metrics like blood pressure and pulse rate. The Apple Watch, for example, can alert users to abnormal cardiac rhythms. Clinical IoMT devices are comparable to consumer IoMT devices, with the exception that they offer a broader sensor selection. Diabetic individuals, for example, can wear glucose monitors to detect changes in their blood sugar levels. Many of these gadgets can establish a connection with a patient's primary care physician, ensuring that the patient receives rapid and accurate treatment.

2.2.3. Community IoMT

Community IoMT refers to the use of IoMT devices across a larger geographical region like a big city. Mobility services, for example, are gadgets that track patients while they are in a car. Outside of the hospital context, paramedics and first responders use emergency response intelligence systems to manage patient parameters. Community IoMT includes technologies that offer remote services in addition to mobile and emergency care. Point-of-care devices, for example, is being used by health care personnel in non-conventional medical venues like a kiosk and schools can be used to distribute medications to patients in locations where traditional infrastructure is inadequate or non-existent. Suppliers may employ IoMT devices in logistics to help with the movement of health care commodities or diagnostic supplies. Sensors, for example, can monitor pressure- or temperature-sensitive shipping containers throughout the transport process to ensure that standards are maintained.

2.2.4. In-Hospital IoMT

Hospitals must monitor the supply and quality of their medical assets throughout time, as well as the movement of staff and patients within the hospital. Health care practitioners track all of these interactions using IoMT sensors and other tracking devices to provide administrators with a clear picture of what is happening.

2.3. Efficient Monitoring and Recording of Information in Real-Time

Modern health care is data-driven. On the other hand, this data will be beneficial only if it is accurate and timely. Misdiagnosis and delivery of the inappropriate treatment have occurred as a result of symptom documentation errors. Doctors used to record information on paper charts, which was the customary method. All of the doctors who would be involved in the patient's treatment would need to get these charts. Charts were more likely to be misplaced when the paper was moved around. For example, if a patient switches doctors or sees a different doctor, such as locum tenens, his or her charts may be lost (Lekkas and Gritzlais, 2007). To keep their records up to date, patients with paper charts relied on their ability to recall their diagnosis and therapy facts.

Patients' test results were also delayed as a result of updating paper records. Patients experienced unnecessarily high levels of anxiety as a result of the extended wait for test results. In modern health care, the process of recording data has improved. Patient information and lab results are entered into a system that is available to a wide range of health care professionals. Furthermore, android devices are used to maintain track of real-time conversations with patients. More precise assessment is now possible because staffs are no longer obliged to transcribe notes, which could lead to mistakes.

The electronic health record (EHR) system from Practice Fusion contains features like centralized chart management, which allows clinicians to access patient records on any device, at any time, and from any location. An EHR system is seen as a crucial component of modern health care since it guarantees that communication with other health care professionals, including such health insurers and diagnostic centres, is retained in one central area. Timely delivery of testing results is also possible with an EHR system. The findings are documented and saved in a database, guaranteeing that they are never lost. The patient may be made aware of the testing results once a doctor has assessed (Hossain et al., 2019).

2.4. Modernized Doctor-Patient Communication

Medical practices should make increasing patient satisfaction a critical objective. The push for patient-centered treatment is a fundamental aspect of modern health care, and doctors must develop new ways to communicate with their patients successfully. Patients should be engaged in ways other than traditional office visits. Health care providers may want to take a cue from other sectors, such as retail, and suggest using chatbots to engage patients on routine issues. Health-care practitioners can create and supervise these chatbots. By guiding patients in the right direction, an online triage system can aid in this type of communication (Noble, 2020).

If chatbots are too advanced for your practice, explore another type of electronic communication that the most of your patients will use. According to a study published in the Journal of the American Board of Family Medicine, communicating with patients via email improved both physician and patient satisfaction. Consider implementing a HIPAA-compliant portal and messaging system, such as Spok, to enable more efficient communication between physician and his patient while maintaining patient confidentiality. Additionally, patients can access information about their medical condition, treatment plans, and test results via communication portals as self-service tools.

Video messaging is another way for medical practitioners to incorporate elements of modern health care into their practice in order to improve communication with their patients. Patients may be familiar with video messaging as a result of their use of social media and messaging applications. Medical professionals can communicate with their patients via video conferencing at a place and time that is convenient for both sides (Parker et al., 2021). Likewise, patients can communicate with their health care provider using videomedicine.com without having to miss work. Offering this level of convenience is thought to result in more excellent continuity of care, higher patient retention, and higher patient satisfaction.

3. Big Data in Modern Health Care System

"Big Data" – Mostly it refers to the huge volume of data that are used to resolve the problems in the real-time. It has got much attention for a decade due to the huge potential it possesses. Many private and public sectors analyze, retain, and produce large amounts of data (Big Data) in order to improve their services. Internet of things devices, medical examination findings, patient medical records, and hospital records are all examples of big data sources in the health care sector. Biomedical research also creates a large amount of big data that is relevant to global health. To extract useful information out of this data, it must be properly maintained and evaluated. Else, resolving a problem through the analysis of massive volume of data is like to searching for a needle in a haystack. Each level of large data processing poses unique obstacles that can be overcome only with the deployment of advanced computer technology for big data analysis. As a result, health care professionals must be properly stocked with the infrastructure necessary to analyze and generate massive volumes of data in order to provide relevant solutions for public health improvement. Effectively managed, processed, and interpreted big data has the potential to change the facet of modern health care by introducing new avenues (Nazir et al., 2020; Neelakandan et al., 2022).

Modern health care organizations may be able to transform medical therapies and customized medicine through a robust integration of biological and health-care data. The workflow of Big Data Analytics in modern day advanced health care is depicted in Figure 4. Large volumes of data are stored in data warehouses from a wide range of sources. These massive amounts of data are analyzed via analytic pipelines in order to identify more prudent and cost-effective health care solutions. A framework of integrating health care analytics and omics data to personalized treatment is depicted in Figure 5. Systematic and integrated omics data analysis in conjunction with health care analytics can boost the development of more precise and individualized treatment solutions. Health care requires sophisticated integration of biomedical data from a variety of sources in order to provide improved medications and patient care. These prospects are so appealing that commercial businesses are currently employing DNA sequences data to help clinicians in generating tailored medical judgments, regardless of the fact that individual genetic data will contain multiple variants. This has the potential to be a game changer for health and medicine in the future (Chen et al., 2020). Due to the particular characteristics of IoMT data, it would demand modified operating software, as well as enhanced hardware and analytic software. In addition, we'd have to handle data from IoMT devices in real-time and evaluate it minute by minute. Health care system personnel are striving to reduce money and improve service quality by utilizing advanced analytics on both internal and external generated data.

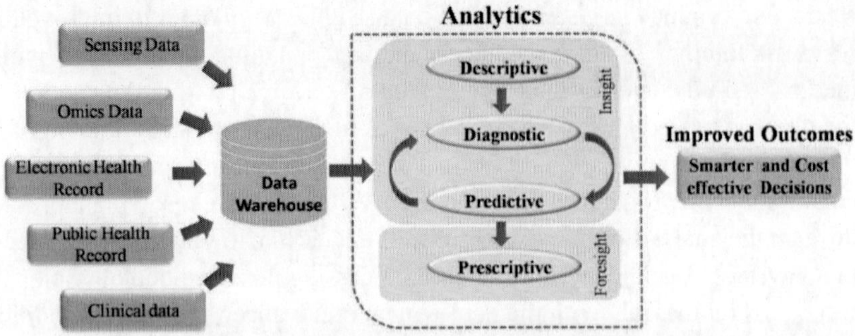

Figure 4. Workflow of Big Data Analytics in Modern Health care.

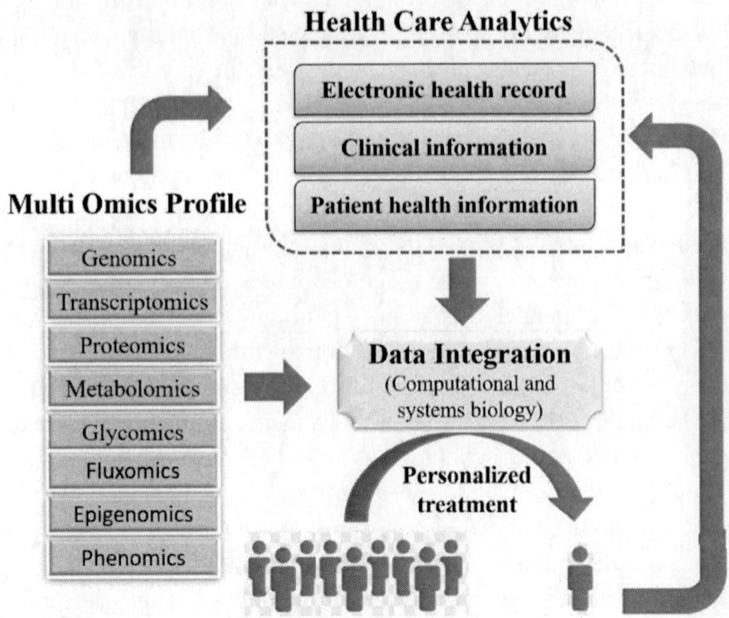

Figure 5. A Framework for Integrating Health care Analytics and Omics Data for Personalized Treatment.

Numerous biological and health care equipment generate a great deal of data, including smartphone applications, mobile biometric sensors, and genomics. As a result, we ought to be conscious of and evaluate what can be actually accomplished with this information. Examining such data, for example, can reveal more information about medical, technical, procedural, and perhaps other areas of health-care improvement. When diverse medical remedies are examined more closely, it appears as though the full extent of patient-specific medical specializations or personalized medicine is being realized. Businesses that provide health care analytics and clinical transformation services contribute to the achievement of more efficient and effective outcomes. These organizations share common goals, including detecting and avoiding big data fraud, establishing platforms for more individualized treatment plans, establishing effective Clinical Decision Support (CDS) tools, and decrease the cost of analytics (Alotaibi et al., 2020). Almost all of them, however, face difficulties from the federal government on the security, sharing, and handling of private data. Despite this, the combined data collection from biomedical researchers and health care organisations has resulted in a proper diagnosis, better knowledge, and helping to treat a wide variety of ailments.

It has also contributed to the establishment of a more robust and sustainable health-care system. The current health care fraternity, which has recognised the potential of big data, has used it in contemporary clinical practices and in modern health care. Computers, ranged from quantum computers to supercomputers, aid in obtaining usable information from a large amount of data in a matter of seconds (Krishna et al., 2021). Despite the infrastructure issues, researchers are delving into large amounts of biomedical data in order to extract useful and novel insights that can improve the existing status of health-care services. Clinical studies, combined pharmacy and insurance claim analytics, and biomarker detection are all part of a novel and creative approach to analyzing vast quantities of electronic health records. The void between unstructured and structured data sources is exploited by big data analytics. The challenge of moving to a unified data environment is well-known. Interestingly, the idea behind big data is that if you have more data, then, the more inferences can be gained and the more projections about future occurrences can be made. Numerous health care companies and renowned consulting firms properly predicted the exponential growth of the big data health care market. Furthermore, in a relatively short period of time, we have seen an explosion in the use of analytics, which has had a profound effect on health care performance and decision-making (Stalin David et al., 2021).

Implementing and integrating a vast volume of medical data obtained across several platforms is a challenge for data scientists. As a result, it is suggested that a health-care revolution is required to integrate health informatics, bioinformatics, and analytics to encourage more tailored and better clinical outcomes. New technologies and strategies need be developed to derive meaningful information from unstructured, semi-structured, and structured data in order to comprehend their nature (unstructured, semi-structured, structured) and complexity (attributes and dimensions). Big data's greatest asset is its inexhaustible potential. The growth and integration of big data has resulted in tremendous advancements in the health care sector over the last several years, ranging from medical data management to drug discovery programs for complex human diseases such as cancer and neurological disorders. Big data will improve health care by enabling the prediction of epidemics (as they relate to people health), the early detection of sickness, and the identification of novel biomarkers and advanced therapeutic involvement strategies for better-quality of life (Ch et al., 2021).

4. Machine Learning in Modern Health Care

Simply explained, Machine Learning (ML) is a type of artificial intelligence in which machines are trained to acquire knowledge without the intervention of humans. The core algorithms in ML are constructed using computational statistics. Computers are fed with data, and the computers then "learn" from it. The information "teaches" "by displaying the computer's intricate patterns and underlying algorithms. The larger the data sample, the more powerful the "machine." ML is becoming more prevalent in health care, where it benefits both patients and clinicians in a variety of ways. The most typical application of ML in health care is to automate medical billing, clinical decision support, and the establishment of clinical care recommendations (Agarwal et al., 2021). ML and health care principles have multiple significant applications in medicine.

The world's first medical ML system capable of anticipating acute toxicities in patients undergoing radiation therapy for head and neck tumours has been developed by MD Anderson researchers. When evaluating images from traditional radiology reports, PET scans, MRI, CT, and radiography, deep learning in health care finds complicated patterns automatically and assists radiologists in making informed decisions. ML-based automatic detection and diagnosis algorithms have been found to perform as well as a skilled physician. For instance, Google's health-care ML algorithms were trained to detect breast cancer and obtained an accuracy of 89 percent, which is generally more accurate than that of radiologists. These are just a few of the numerous ML applications in health care.

Almost 80% of the data stored in electronic health record systems is unstructured health care data suitable for ML. These are documents or text files, not data fragments that previously could not be inspected without the assistance of a human. Human language, also referred to as "natural language," is very intricate, devoid of regularity, and replete with vagueness, jargon, and ambiguity. Natural language processing (NLP) tools are frequently used in health care to convert these papers into more valuable and analyzable data. The majority of NLP-based deep learning applications in health care require the use of medical ML (Iroju and Olaleke, 2015).

One of the top ML for Health care applications is a bot system that significantly reduces treatment time. A virtual nurse acts as a voice-activated health care assistant for patients, delivering information on a medication, variety of disorders, and health problems. If a patient requires immediate assistance and travelling to the doctor is impossible, an AI assistant can be quite useful. Data engineers are developing solutions for all medical tasks involving overall health monitoring and assisting in the cure or prevention of disease.

However, the machine does not perform all tasks. For example, machine learning data must be arranged so that the computer can detect patterns and conclusions more quickly. It is usually done by people who use annotations over the input to tag elements of the dataset. This function is filled by clinical specialists who also evaluate data, design new rules, and optimize machine performance. However, in order for health care machine learning algorithms to train quickly and successfully, the data annotations must be accurate and relevant to our goal of extracting vital ideas with appropriate context (Tvardik et al., 2018).

There are numerous ML algorithms explained in the literature. Each algorithm is unique and applied to specific conditions. The performance of the ML algorithm mainly depends upon the training data and its precision (Jain et al., 2020; Raj and Balaji, 2021). These algorithms can be used for pattern recognition, classification, natural language processing. Figure 6 depicts the various machine learning algorithm and their detailed classification.

Artificial Neural Networks are the most common ML algorithms used in health care. For example, CNN (convolutional neural networks) are used to do picture recognition, detection, and identification. These are a sophisticated system of artificial neuron layers that have been pre-trained on images of injured cells in order to "remember" the appearances of harming cells. These medical specialties are particularly challenging for data scientists to crack since they need the most difficult branch of ML, including deep learning. However, it enables the creation of neural networks and the detection of organism-harming cells (like cancer cells).

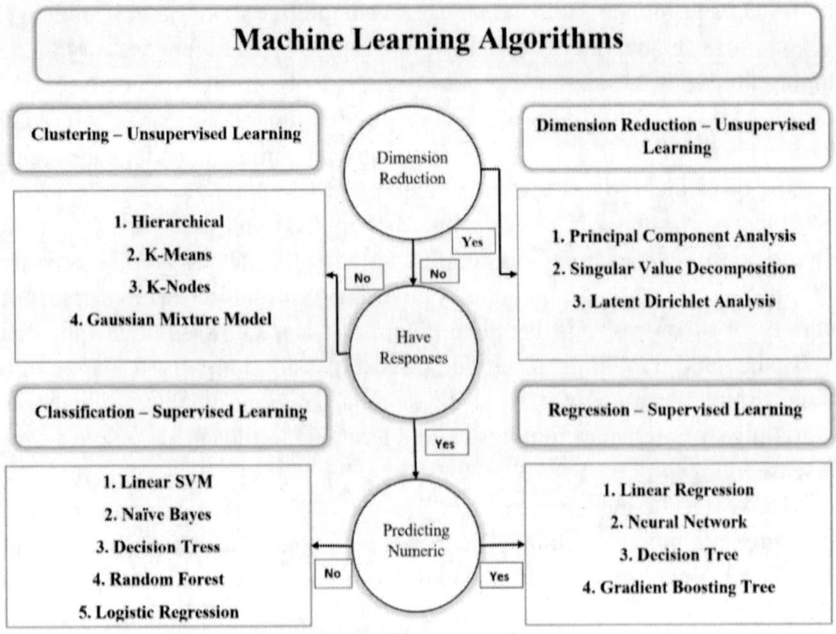

Figure 6. Classification of Machine Learning Algorithms.

ML in health care technology searches for cancer-affected cells with an accuracy comparable to that of a qualified doctor in oncology. The ability of ML to assess organic fluids from patients (such as tissues, urine, and blood) can boost a pathologist's capacity to evaluate them. In comparison to an automated model, human vision using a microscope performs analysis at a rate of about half that of an automated model. As a result, installing CNN-based patient diagnostic applications can assist hospitals and research centers (Ke et al., 2020). Additionally, we must accept that we continue to face a knowledge gap about the causes of unusual diseases and the relationship between these diseases and the characteristics of those who are afflicted. In this vein, certain ML in Health care firms contribute to the market by creating novel methods for analyzing and tracking information extracted from patient images.

As smart medical devices grow more common, technology-enabled health care is becoming a reality. The health care business embraces innovation, which is why AI's future in health care is highly promising. For instance, Google recently unveiled an algorithm that accurately diagnoses breast cancer in mammograms, and Stanford University researchers employed Deep Learning to detect skin cancer. Among other things, artificial intelligence is responsible for analyzing millions of different data points and effectively anticipating risks and outcomes.

The various other important machine learning applications in modern health care are a. Disease Identification and Diagnosis, b. Artificial Intelligence assisted Surgery, c. Epidemic Control, d. Leveraging Medical Data, e. Clinical Trial Improvement and Medical Research, f. Personalizing Treatment, g. Image Analysis, h. Improvement in Health Records.

4.1. Disease Identification and Diagnosis

ML is extremely successful at diagnosing; indeed, it is one of the most effective fields. Numerous types of cancer and genetic disorders are difficult to diagnose, but machine learning may be able to detect most of the cases in their early stages. Watson Genomics from IBM is a great example of this. This program combines genome-wide tumour sequencing and cognitive computing to expedite cancer detection. Additionally, P1vital's PReDicT (Predicting Response to Depression Treatment) initiative aims to build a feasible technique for utilizing artificial intelligence to enhance diagnosis and treatment in traditional hospitals.

Diabetes is a highly prevalent and sometimes dangerous condition. This not only wreaks havoc on a person's health, but it also contributes to the onset of a plethora of other significant illnesses. Diabetic renal disease, heart disease, and nerve damage are the most common complications. Machine Learning could aid in the early detection of diabetes, perhaps saving lives. KNN, Decision Tree, and Naive Bayes are examples of classification algorithms that could develop a diabetes prediction system. In terms of performance and calculation time, Naive Bayes is the most efficient (Harimoorthy and Thangavelu, 2021).

When it comes to metabolism, the liver is one of the most essential organs in the human body. Chronic hepatitis, liver cancer, and cirrhosis are all disorders that can affect it (Allen et al., 2018). It's difficult to anticipate liver illness using massive volumes of medical data accurately, but there have already been some notable advances. The distinction is made through machine learning methods such as classification and clustering.

Another great use of Machine Learning is in the early stages of drug research for patients. For instance, Microsoft's Project Hanover is presently utilizing AI-based technologies to identify personalized drug combinations to treat Acute Myeloid Leukemia.

4.2. Artificial Intelligence Assisted Surgery

It is perhaps the most important use of Machine Learning, and it will grow in popularity in the near future. The following are the several types of robotic Surgery: Surgical competence assessment, robotic surgical material improvement, surgical workflow modelling, and automatic suturing. Suturing is the process of closing an open wound. Making this technique computerized shortens the Surgery while relieving the surgeon of stress. Even though it is too early to talk of robots performing entirely surgical procedures, they may now aid and assist a doctor in manipulating surgical gear. It is predicted to grow to a special industry with a 39 billion dollars capital in the following five years. When a medical operation is carried out, the robot's robotic hands will be used to assist the doctor in grabbing tools (Rimmer et al., 2021). This type of procedure reduces surgical problems by 50% and cuts the amount of time a patient spends in the operating room by 20%. While collecting data on each AI Surgery, ML algorithms for health care data analytics also assess and identify new procedure opportunities.

4.3. Epidemic Control

In 2021, experts will have access to data analytics from video feeds, news websites, social media trends, and satellites. It might be processed by neural networks, which could draw inferences about epidemic outbreaks throughout the world. Before they cause widespread havoc, threatening ailments could be stopped in their tracks. It is especially crucial in Third World nations, where advanced medical systems are lacking (Mooris et al., 2021). Since it is a World wide web-based reporting network that supervises pandemic reports from all around the world, ProMED-mail is likely the best example of this field. Artificial Intelligence is also widely used in assisting in the prevention of epidemic disease on farms and food safety.

4.4. Leveraging Medical Data

Investigators nowadays have significant exposure to a vast volume of data that patients have made available to the public. It will be the source of future advancements in Machine Learning in Medicine. The development in Big Data and Data Mining techniques makes it easier and more efficient. Medtronic and IBM have already collaborated on understanding, collecting, and making public real-time insulin data. There will be even more possibilities as the Internet of Things (IoT) develops. Additionally, public data will aid in patient diagnostics and the issuance of medication prescriptions (Kumar and Tripathi, 2021).

4.5. Clinical Trial Improvement and Medical Research

Clinical studies can take years to complete and involve considerable financial inputs. Based on criteria such as a person's social media activity or history of doctor visits, machine learning can provide predictive analytics to discover the appropriate prospects for clinical studies. The technology may also recommend the appropriate sample sizes to test, reducing the number of data-based errors.

4.6. Personalizing Treatment

Medicine is making remarkable strides with machine learning. IBM Watson Oncology stands out as a pioneer in this field, offering various therapy options based on a patient's medical history. Things will get even better when establishing tailored treatment regimens as improved biosensors become more widely available, offering more data for algorithms. Somatix, a business-to-business-to-consumer company, has developed an application that monitors the unconscious behaviors we engage in on a daily basis and notifies us to those that may be detrimental in the long run.

4.7. Image Analysis

With its InnerEye project, Microsoft is transforming health care data analysis. Computer Vision is used by this startup to evaluate medical images in order to diagnose and treat. It is becoming more well-known in the field of health care analytics software as technology advances. Machine Learning will become more efficient soon, allowing for analyzing even more data points to establish an automatic diagnosis (Priya and Rakinikanth, 2021; Qureshi et al., 2021; Kishor and Chakraborty, 2021; Guo et al., 2015).

4.8. Improvement in Health Records

Despite all of these technological advancements, maintaining health data remains a pain. While it is significantly faster now, it still takes a long time. Vector machines and machine learning-based techniques to OCR recognition could be utilized to classify documents. Two noteworthy examples are MathWorks' machine learning-based handwriting recognition system and Google's Cloud Vision API.

Conclusion

In recent years, countries all around the world have spent enormous sums of money on health care. The current pandemic emergency has pushed it to new heights. Sensor and wireless technology improvements and their integration into the traditional health care system have made it more advanced and user-friendlier. In recent years, a variety of implanted and wearable sensor devices have been developed. The vital signs of the person who wears or implants these devices can be continuously checked utilizing these gadgets. The Internet of Medical Things (IoMT) is a network of medical equipment and hardware linked together. It allows for real-time monitoring of a person's condition, even from a rural location. The continual sensing and monitoring of these indicators generate a massive amount of data in the data repository. The current breakthroughs in Big Data and its use in the modern health care system make managing these massive amounts of data feasible and simple. The useful information can be extracted from the raw data utilizing these strategies. Multiple machine learning algorithms can be used to anticipate the patient's current status and future occurrence from this data. The current effort delves into the architecture of several wearable monitoring and tracking devices. It also goes over the different IoMT settings. The acquisition of medical data and the use of Big Data to better manage it can also be explained in detail. There are numerous examples of various Machine Learning algorithms applied in disease prediction and detection. All of this leads us to conclude that incorporating IoMT, wearable or implantable sensor devices, Big Data, and Machine Learning into modern health care makes it superior to traditional health care and more user-friendly.

References

Agarwal, P., Ch, M. A., Kharate, D. S., Raj, E. F. I., & Balamuralitharan, S. (2021). Parameter Estimation of COVID-19 Second Wave BHRP Transmission Model by Using Principle Component Analysis. *Annals of the Romanian Society for Cell Biology*, 446-457.

Ahmad, M. A., Eckert, C., & Teredesai, A. (2018, August). Interpretable machine learning in health care. In *Proceedings of the 2018 ACM international conference on bioinformatics, computational biology, and health informatics* (pp. 559-560).

Allen, A. M., Van Houten, H. K., Sangaralingham, L. R., Talwalkar, J. A., & McCoy, R. G. (2018). Health care cost and utilization in nonalcoholic fatty liver disease: real-world data from a large US claims database. *Hepatology*, *68*(6), 2230-2238.

Alotaibi, S., Mehmood, R., Katib, I., Rana, O., & Albeshri, A. (2020). Sehaa: A big data analytics tool for health care symptoms and diseases detection using Twitter, Apache Spark, and Machine Learning. *Applied Sciences*, *10*(4), 1398.

Ch, G., Jana, S., Majji, S., Kuncha, P., & Tigadi, A. (2021). Diagnosis of COVID-19 using 3D CT scans and vaccination for COVID-19. *World Journal of Engineering*.

Chen, P. T., Lin, C. L., & Wu, W. N. (2020). Big data management in health care: Adoption challenges and implications. *International Journal of Information Management*, *53*, 102078.

Datta, S., Barua, R., & Das, J. (2020). Application of artificial intelligence in modern health care system. *Alginates—recent uses of this natural polymer*.

Stalin David, D., Nageswara Rao, G., Swain, M. P., Venkatesh, U. S., Fantin Irudaya Raj, E., & Saravanan, D. (2021). Inflammatory syndrome experiments related with COVID-19. Turkish Journal of Physiotherapy and Rehabilitation, 765-768.

Gope, P., Gheraibia, Y., Kabir, S., & Sikdar, B. (2020). A secure IoT-based modern health care system with fault-tolerant decision making process. *IEEE Journal of Biomedical and Health Informatics*, *25*(3), 862-873.

Guo, L., Yang, J. J., Peng, L., Li, J., & Liang, Q. (2015). A computer-aided health care system for cataract classification and grading based on fundus image analysis. *Computers in Industry*, *69*, 72-80.

Harimoorthy, K., & Thangavelu, M. (2021). Multi-disease prediction model using improved SVM-radial bias technique in health care monitoring system. *Journal of Ambient Intelligence and Humanized Computing*, *12*(3), 3715-3723.

Hossain, A., Quaresma, R., & Rahman, H. (2019). Investigating factors influencing the physicians' adoption of electronic health record (EHR) in health care system of Bangladesh: An empirical study. *International Journal of Information Management*, *44*, 76-87.

Hung, K., Zhang, Y. T., & Tai, B. (2004, September). Wearable medical devices for tele-home health care. In *The 26th Annual International Conference of the IEEE Engineering in Medicine and Biology Society* (Vol. 2, pp. 5384-5387). IEEE.

Iroju, O. G., & Olaleke, J. O. (2015). A systematic review of natural language processing in health care. *International Journal of Information Technology and Computer Science*, *7*(8), 44-50.

Jain, D., Sangale, D. M. D., & Raj, E. (2020). A Pilot Survey Of Machine Learning Techniques In Smart Grid Operations Of Power Systems. *European Journal of Molecular & Clinical Medicine*, *7*(7), 203-210.

Ke, H., Chen, D., Shah, T., Liu, X., Zhang, X., Zhang, L., & Li, X. (2020). Cloud-aided online EEG classification system for brain health care: A case study of depression evaluation with a lightweight CNN. *Software: Practice and Experience*, *50*(5), 596-610.

Khan, J. Y., Yuce, M. R., Bulger, G., & Harding, B. (2012). Wireless body area network (WBAN) design techniques and performance evaluation. *Journal of medical systems*, *36*(3), 1441-1457.

Khan, Y., Ostfeld, A. E., Lochner, C. M., Pierre, A., & Arias, A. C. (2016). Monitoring of vital signs with flexible and wearable medical devices. *Advanced materials*, *28*(22), 4373-4395.

Kishor, A., & Chakraborty, C. (2021). Artificial intelligence and internet of things based health care 4.0 monitoring system. *Wireless Personal Communications*, 1-17.

Krishna, B., Amuthavalli, G., StalinDavid, D., Raj, E. F., & Saravanan, D. (2021). Certain Investigation of SARS-COVID-2-Induced Kawasaki-Like Disease in Indian Youngsters. *Annals of the Romanian Society for Cell Biology*, 1167-1182.

Kumar, R., & Tripathi, R. (2021). Towards design and implementation of security and privacy framework for internet of medical things (iomt) by leveraging blockchain and ipfs technology. *The Journal of Supercomputing*, 1-40.

Lekkas, D., & Gritzalis, D. (2007). Long-term verifiability of the electronic health care records' authenticity. *International journal of medical informatics*, *76*(5-6), 442-448.

Morris, D. H., Rossine, F. W., Plotkin, J. B., & Levin, S. A. (2021). Optimal, near-optimal, and robust epidemic control. *Communications Physics*, *4*(1), 1-8.

Nazir, S., Khan, S., Khan, H. U., Ali, S., García-Magariño, I., Atan, R. B., & Nawaz, M. (2020). A comprehensive analysis of health care big data management, analytics and scientific programming. *IEEE Access*, *8*, 95714-95733.

Neelakandan, S., Rene Beulah, J., Prathiba, L., Murthy, G. L. N., Irudaya Raj, E. F., & Arulkumar, N. (2022). Blockchain with deep learning-enabled secure health care data transmission and diagnostic model. *International Journal of Modeling, Simulation, and Scientific Computing,* 2241006.

Noble, L. M. (2020). Doctor-patient communication and adherence to treatment. In *Adherence to treatment in medical conditions* (pp. 51-82). CRC Press.

Parker, L., Ryan, R., Young, S., & Hill, S. (2021). Medications and doctor–patient communication. *Aust J Gen Pract*, *50*(10), 709-14.

Priya, E., & Rajinikanth, V. (2021). *Signal and Image Processing Techniques for the Development of Intelligent Health care Systems*. Singapore: Springer.

Pustokhina, I. V., Pustokhin, D. A., Gupta, D., Khanna, A., Shankar, K., & Nguyen, G. N. (2020). An effective training scheme for deep neural network in edge computing enabled Internet of medical things (IoMT) systems. *IEEE Access*, *8*, 107112-107123.

Qureshi, F., & Krishnan, S. (2018). Wearable hardware design for the internet of medical things (IoMT). *Sensors*, *18*(11), 3812.

Qureshi, K. N., Alhudhaif, A., Ali, M., Qureshi, M. A., & Jeon, G. (2021). Self-assessment and deep learning-based coronavirus detection and medical diagnosis systems for health care. *Multimedia Systems*, 1-10.

Raj, E. F. I., & Balaji, M. (2021). Analysis and classification of faults in switched reluctance motors using deep learning neural networks. *Arabian Journal for Science and Engineering*, *46*(2), 1313-1332.

Rimmer, L., Howard, C., Picca, L., & Bashir, M. (2021). The automaton as a surgeon: the future of artificial intelligence in emergency and general surgery. *European Journal of Trauma and Emergency Surgery*, *47*(3), 757-762.

Stawicki, S. P., Green, A. M., Lu, G. G., Domer, G., Oskin, T., & Firstenberg, M. S. (2019). Introductory Chapter: patient safety is the cornerstone of modern health care delivery systems. *Vignettes in Patient Safety*, *4*, 1-11.

Tvardik, N., Kergourlay, I., Bittar, A., Segond, F., Darmoni, S., & Metzger, M. H. (2018). Accuracy of using natural language processing methods for identifying health care-associated infections. *International journal of medical informatics*, *117*, 96-102.

Yu, K. H., Beam, A. L., & Kohane, I. S. (2018). Artificial intelligence in health care. *Nature biomedical engineering*, *2*(10), 719-731.

Chapter 8

Real-Time Intelligent Application for Lifestyle and Mind State Monitoring and Simulation Using Digital Twin, Artificial Intelligence and IoT

Nayana Gupta*, N. Manoj Kumar† and Deepak Kumar Bagchi‡
Coforge, Bengaluru, Karnataka, India

Abstract

A worldwide health catastrophe has resulted from the pandemic, which has had a profound influence on how we see our daily lives. On one side we have witnessed the lack of medical facilities which has generated a lot of fear in people's minds. On the other side, there has been exponential growth towards awareness of self-health. People are more interested in knowing how their body is reacting. Also, there has been a growing focus on mental health. This shift has motivated researchers and practitioners to understand and perceive a solution that can simulate the lifestyle using routine data. Further, this leads to an important addition in the space of personalized lifestyle tracker applications. Cutting-edge technologies AI and IoT with Digital Twins will shift the current monitoring and treatment selection based on the state of the patient of today to an optimized state of the patient of tomorrow. This would be a

*Corresponding Author's Email: er.nayana.g@gmail.com.
†Corresponding Author's Email: manojkumarkpn1192@gmail.com.
‡Corresponding Author's Email: deepakbagchi@yahoo.com.

In: AI-Enabled IoT for Smart Health Care Systems
Editors: Tawseef Ayoub Shaikh, Tabasum Rasool and Mohammed Wasid
ISBN: 978-1-68507-977-2

key part of the P4-Medicine – predictive, preventive, personalized, and participative.

Each of us is so unique in many ways that most of the current treatments conceived for the "average patient" are highly inefficient to the "actual patient." Given the significant influence of routine on a person's health, this study first broadens the typical input sources currently used by such applications. The idea was to generate a wholesome analysis of the human lifestyle and mental state. The work divides the lifestyle into four major parts (Meal intake, Physical activities, Digital Medium Interaction (Digital Screen interaction), and Social activities). These data points are collected using multiple different IoT devices (open-sourced and customized), for example, smaller wearables (sensors, watches), mobile usage trackers, laptop usage trackers, medication trackers, food trackers, and so on. Also, we have designed a smaller set of questions to evaluate cognitive and social behavior. This information is then fed in real-time to the digital twin. Using the above data, multiple simulation experiments have been conducted for multiple lifestyle parameters to predict future lifestyle state (Energized, Active, Normal, Lazy, and Indisposed) and mind state (Happy, Calm, Sensitive, Sad, and Stressed). This work further considers medical staff and other types of users to evaluate how the score is going to improve parameters like decision time for treatment, better availability of alternatives, and optimization of monitoring time.

We understand that this solution is helpful for personal usage as well as for medical staff (doctors/nursing staff). This can help people track their health concerns such as heart disease, diabetes, pregnancy, mental health, and others. It will inspire people to live healthier lifestyles. This will also make it easier for family members and nursing staff to remotely discuss and report on a patient's health information, as well as keep track of prescriptions. Using a Digital twin interface, Doctors can simulate the patient's health parameters and get predictions based on his/her past health history. It will allow doctors to determine the personalized treatment for the patient and enable cost reductions at hospitals through efficiency optimizations.

Keywords: digital twin, artificial intelligence, Internet of Things (IoT), classification, health care, lifestyle

1. Introduction

1.1. Background

It has been recorded from recent surveys and many other article and blogs which are available all over the internet that people are very much aware of the overall health and they want to take care of their health now, be it physical or mental.

On the other hand, this is also noticed that there are multiple different ways available to track and monitor one's health, like using Fitbit devices, fitness bands, using mobile apps to track phone usage, meditation – yoga apps, etc. Also, many IT companies use laptop usage software's to track the activities of the employees on the laptop or Desktop.

We understand a fed of a solution that can track, monitor, predict and prescribe to the users based on multiple activities. These activities would include different activities from his full day. For example, physical activities through fitness band, mobile usage activities through mobile apps tracking app, laptop usage from the activity logs.

Here for this chapter, we have combined and brought together these different apps with IoT and AI, to provide an overall lifestyle tracker solution to the user.

1.2. Motivation

Physical and Mental health awareness has increased in the past few years and specifically after Covid-19. Many health care initiatives, awareness projects, and fitness enterprises are on the horizon. People themselves are very much aware and willing to put effort into a better lifestyle. Work from home phenomena has affected the lifestyle of working professionals widely. This has inspired us to explore the overall health of working professionals and identify the strongest predictors of physical and mind state.

Also, some questions that popped up and seemed worth exploring are:

1. What all different parameters affect the human lifestyle over a period of time?
2. How is digital media usage affecting the lifestyle?
3. How does mobile/laptop usage affect lifestyle and mental state?

4. What is the frequency of common mental health disorders like anxiety?
5. What are the strongest predictors of mental health illness?
6. Can these all be combined together and utilized for leading a better life?

2. Literature Review

As we were doing the literature reviews, our motivation was growing more. It helped us mainly in identifying the data points.

On the one hand, the entire world is dealing with the COVID-19 pandemic, which has also had an impact on the mental health of millions of people. According to WHO, approximately 7.5% of Indians suffer from some form of mental disorder in 2020, and by the end of this year, approximately 20% of India will suffer from mental illnesses. According to statistics, 56 million Indians suffer from depression, with another 38 million suffering from anxiety disorders [1]. Below Figure 1 is a screenshot of 2016 NHMS report, where WP is weighted percentage of people in India:

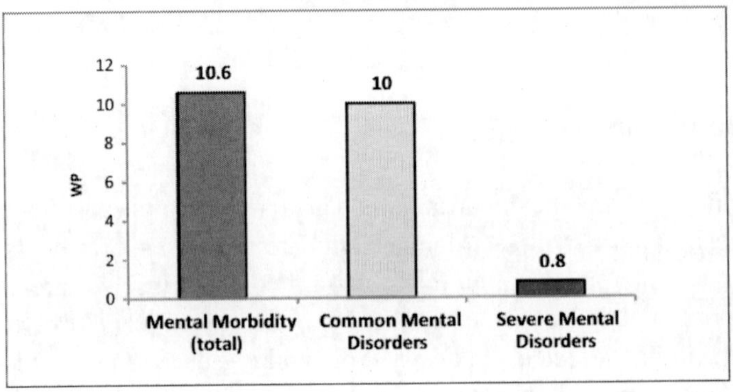

Figure 1. NMHS survey 2016.

Depression, anxiety disorders, and substance use disorders are among the most common mental disorders (CMDs), affecting nearly 10% of the population. This group of disorders is also closely linked to the causes and consequences of several non - communicable disease (NCD), contributing to a significantly increased health burden. Previously, these disorders went unnoticed in the planning and delivery of health-care programmes. Individuals and families also disregard and ignore these disorders until they become severe [2].

India's digital journey has been growing stronger. In 2020, the country had the world's second-largest internet population, with over 749 million users. 744 million of these users accessed the internet through their mobile phones. Estimates suggest that by 2040, this figure will have risen to more than 1.5 billion [3]. This has had a significant impact on the adoption of health and fitness apps, and will continue to do so in the future.

According to App Annie, a mobile and data analytics firm, there were 20% more downloads in the health and fitness categories on iOS and Google Play in March 2021 than the previous month. From March 2021 benchmarks, HealthifyMe, a health and fitness app, had a 15% boost in new user installations, as well as a 20% increase in previous users reinstalling and returning to the app. The app is mostly used by people between the ages of 21 and 45, who devote 35 minutes every day on it. [4] Similar stories can be found for other apps, including meditation apps.

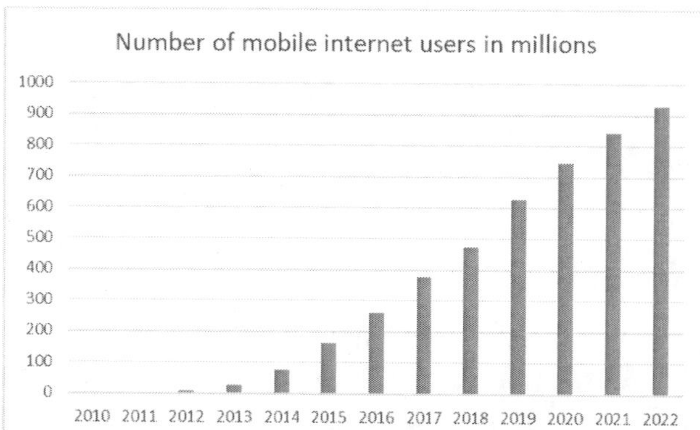

Figure 2. Number of mobile internet users in millions [3].

An era of investing in a fitness band started few years back that constantly monitors your body's vitals and also encourages you to inculcate one good habit at a time and helps achieve your fitness goals timely. With advancements, now user can monitor SpO2 levels, heart rate, sleep, stress, steps and calories burnt etc.

Few other claims from health organizations and researches:

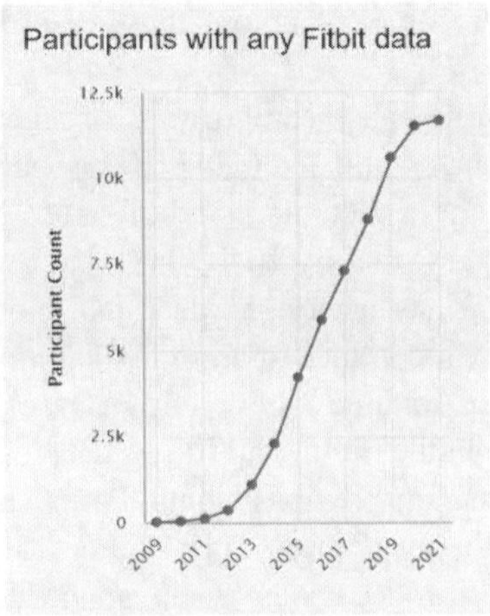

Figure 3. Participants with any Fitbit data over years [6].

- Scoring 150 heart points each week can help live longer, sleep better and boost the mood. (American Heart Association).
- In recent years, there has been much debate about the potential benefits of walking 10,000 steps per day, with some attempting to claim that it is not as beneficial to your health as people have been persuaded.
- Google Fit will encourage users to focus on the amount of time they spend exercising each day, instead of the number of steps they keep taking.
- Google has joined hands with the World Health Organization (WHO) and the American Heart Association (AHA) to introduce two major activity goals in the new Google Fit update, which is available on Android and the Wear OS smartwatch. Move Minutes and Heart Points are the references of these new features.
- Move Minutes will be used to track the amount of time one spends doing physical activity, which will include small acts like taking the stairs or going for a walk.

Many factors interact to influence the health of individuals and communities. The circumstances and environment in which people live determine whether or not they are healthy. Where we live, the state of our environment, genetics, our income, education level, and our relationships with friends and family all have a significant impact on our health. More typically regarded issues such as health care availability and affordability, on the other hand, have a significantly less impact [5].

The social and economic environment, the physical environment, and a person's fundamental characteristics and behavioural patterns are all determinants of health.

We have come to the realization that simply displaying statistics is not going to be enough. We wanted a solution that could both forecast and prescribe improvements for the future.

Prescriptive analytics is a branch of data analytics that focuses on prescribing viable remedies to a problem. It evaluates historical and real-time data and makes future predictions using modelling, data mining, and artificial intelligence. It provides health care organisations with a variety of "what if" scenarios to compare in order to discover the best potential answer for the patient, or in our case, the regular user.

3. Methodology

3.1. System Architecture

3.1.1. Data Sources

- Smartwatch: It gathers sensor information (Accelerometer, Gyroscope, Infrared, and Heart rate sensor) at indicated and adjustable frequencies and computes a wide scope of proactive tasks, for example, Heart rate, Oxygen saturation, Stress, Step, Calories, Distance, Activity, and Sleep.
- Mobile App usage: Data on Daily use of Mobile is accumulated by installing "Application Usage - Manage/Track Usage" to the mobile from the Google Play store. It gives the following highlights

  1. App usage history: collect the time spent on each app by the user
  2. Check phone history: collect the number of times the user locked and unlocked his or her phone
  3. Activity history: collect the amount of time the user spends using apps
  4. Location history: show the apps that a user accessed at a specific location

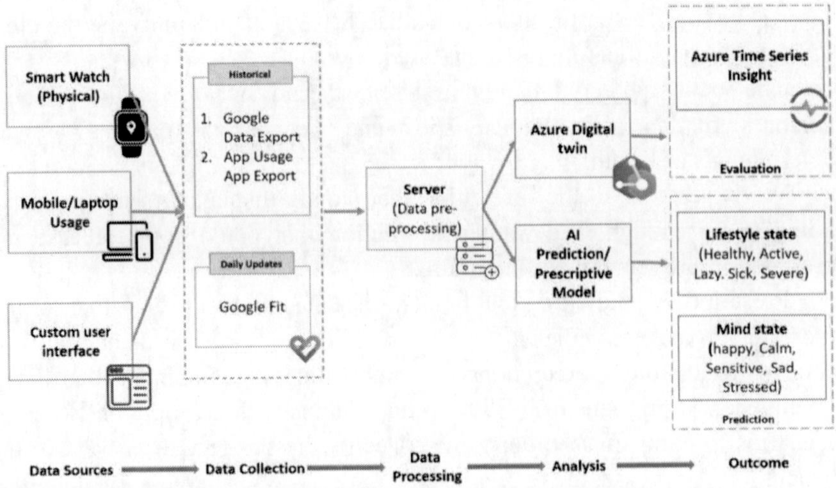

Figure 4. System Architecture.

5. Notification history: display the moment when apps sent out notifications
6. Battery history: show a graph of battery usage
7. Over-use reminder: when a person spends too much time on their phone or apps, it will be reminded
8. Lock mode: PIN-protect app settings and overuse reminder options
9. Most used apps – widgets or a notice that shows the most frequently used apps
10. Track all installs: keeps track of all the apps that the user installed or uninstalled
11. App install reminder: Notifications when apps are installed, as well as a daily summary of installed apps
12. Manage apps: Apps can be uninstalled with a single tap, and apps can be sorted by a variety of criteria

- Custom user interface: User interface is used to feed non-synced smartwatch data (Stress, Sp02, Sleep) and daily parameters (Laptop usage and personal questions) manually to the system one time per day. The below image shows the Custom User interface Screen.

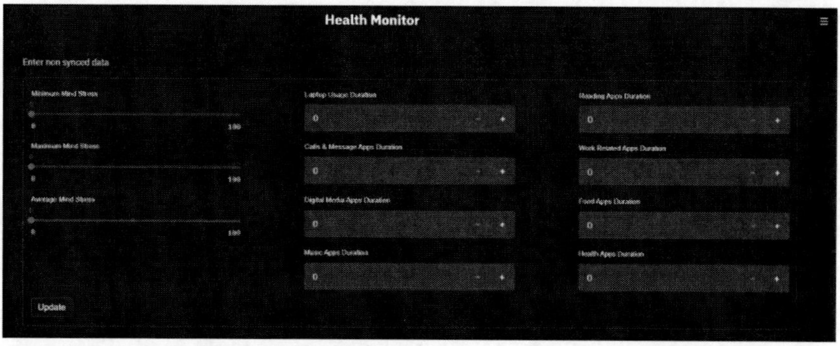

Figure 5. Custom User interface Screen.

3.2. Data Collection and Transmission

The system collects sensor data primarily from Smartwatch, Mobile App, and Custom user interface. Calculated Smartwatch data will be synced with the smartwatch mobile app whenever it is connected to Mobile Bluetooth v5.0. The Smartwatch app will send the synchronized data to the Google Fit server over a Wi-Fi or 4G network connection. Google Fit platform will analyze all the data available from different sources and merge it logically. For example, a person's Step count tracked in both smartwatch and mobile is collected, stored in respective Google Fit Data Sources. The step counts available in the smartwatch data source and mobile data source are merged to get the most complete step count. When merging data, watch data is prioritized over phone data, it avoids counting duplicate steps. When the Data Type is read by the Google Fit Client (Rest API/Python SDK), The Google Fit platform returns the accurate merged information. Data Collection is performed in two ways as follows

- Historical Data collection: Google Fit has a variety of health data that was collected by smartphones across months or even years, and the platform frequently backs it up. The Google Fit platform frequently takes the backup of it. This historical data can be downloaded from Google Fit in minutes using "Google's data export tool" by signing in to the Google Takeout website [7]. Google Fit provides an option to download both Activities data and the daily summaries of user's sessions. The data export process can be customized to export at once or by scheduling automatic exports every two months along with File Type and File Size. Mobile Apps Usage data is exported by installing

App Usage [8] application from the Play store. It provides an option to Export Usage history, Activity history, Daily usage, Check device history, Notification history, Install history, Battery history, Location history, and Apps list as CSV Files for the specified duration.

- Daily Data collection: Sensor readings collected in Mobile and smartwatch are ingested to Google Fit Platform over Wi-Fi connection or Cellular, which allows storing of collected data on the server for real-time or Daily visualization and analysis. Google Fit Platform stores the Synced Data to its respective Data Sources. For example, Step Count Data is collected and stored in the Data Source named "com.google.step_count.delta" and so on. Non-Synced Data is captured by a Custom user interface daily. Google Fit Platform supports storing Custom Data. As per the requirements of data storage, custom data sources are created through REST APIs and returned Data Stream IDs are noted for future usage. Data is posted to the Google Fit Platform via the Google Fit Python Client, which bypasses Data Stream IDs and uses the HTTPS communication protocol to assure data security. For Example, Laptop Usage is captured by creating a custom data source named "com.custom.laptop.usage." Updated Google Fit Data is retrieved in the server using Google Fit Platform REST APIs and Python Client SDK. Retrieved data is preprocessed and converted into interpretable variables.

3.3. Data Preprocessing

Phone app usage data is bundled based on the functioning and intent of different apps as shown below:

Some of the Fitness band data points are discarded. Below is the final list of derived columns:

4. Analysis

This is divided into 3 parts:

1. Digital Twins Modeling

- Data Explained in Table 1 is digitally represented as real-world things using Azure Digital Twins. Microsoft Azure cloud offers Digital Twins Service. Azure Digital Twins is an Internet of Things (IoT) platform as a service (PaaS) to create comprehensive models of the physical environment, provide relationships and interactions between people, spaces, and devices. Azure Digital Twins work with Azure data analytics and AI services to let users track past events and forecast future ones. The data set is divided into six Digital twins (Heart, Mind, Laptop, MobileApps, Movement, and Lifestyle) in order to produce a digital duplicate of physical parameters that influence human health.

Table 1. Mobile Apps grouped into different functions

Call_Message	DigitalMedia	Music	Reading	WorkRelated	Food	Health
Zoom	Instagram	Gaana	Dainik Bhaskar	Gmail	Swiggy	StepSetGo
Call	Facebook	Wynk Music	Google News	Outlook	Zomato	Fit
Phone	YouTube	Amazon Music	Kindle	Teams	Dominos	Home Workout
Contacts	Twitter		Inshorts			
Contacts and dialer	LinkedIn		Apple News			
Messaging	Amazon		Daily Hunt			
WhatsApp	Prime Video					
Snapchat	discovery+					
Messages	Netflix					
Telegram	Flipkart					
Messenger	ZEE5					
Messaging	Sharechat					
Duo						

- Azure Digital Twins provide an open modeling language using a JSON-LD based language called Digital Twin Definition Language (DTDL) that can be used to develop custom domain models of any physical devices. A model is like a class in an object – oriented programming language which defines a data shape of physical device or concept in the real work environment. DTDL is programming-language independent. DTDL version 2 is now used by Azure Digital Twins. A DTDL model interface contains Property (represent the state of an entity), Telemetry (represent measurements or events/sensor readings), Relationship (represent how twin is connected with other twins), component (build model interfaces as an assembly of other interfaces). Figure 6 shows how the data set columns are grouped into 5 Digital twins. Multiple instances can be created for each Model. The Azure Digital Twin Explorer is used to upload these models. Figure 7: Shows the Model Graph in Azure Digital Twin Explorer. Example of Heart model is represented in DTDL as follows:

Table 2. Derived columns from raw data

Data Columns	Data Source	Historical Data Source	Daily Data Source	Data Source ID
PersonID				
Date	Derived			
Day				
Call_Message	Android App(App Usage - Manage/Track Usage)	App Usage - Manage/Track Usage Export	Google Fit Activity Rest API	raw:com.custom.mobile.apps:292824132082:custom:model1:mobile2abs
DigitalMedia				raw:com.custom.mobile.apps:292824132082:custom:model1:mobile2abs
Music				raw:com.custom.mobile.apps:292824132082:custom:model1:mobile2abs
Reading				raw:com.custom.mobile.apps:292824132082:custom:model1:mobile2abs
WorkRelated				raw:com.custom.mobile.apps:292824132082:custom:model1:mobile2abs
Food				raw:com.custom.mobile.apps:292824132082:custom:model1:mobile2abs
Health				raw:com.custom.mobile.apps:292824132082:custom:model1:mobile2abs
Total				Derived
LaptopUsage	Smart Watch Synced with Google Fit	Google Fit Activity Export		raw:com.custom.laptop.usage:292824132082:custom:model1:a1fage35
Average heart rate (bpm)				derived:com.google.heart_rate.bpm:com.google.android.gms:merge_heart_rate_bpm
Max heart rate (bpm)				derived:com.google.heart_rate.bpm:com.google.android.gms:merge_heart_rate_bpm
Min heart rate (bpm)				derived:com.google.heart_rate.bpm:com.google.android.gms:merge_heart_rate_bpm
Average Blood Oxygen(%)				raw:com.google.oxygen_saturation:com.google.android.apps.fitness:user_input
Heart Points				derived:com.google.heart_minutes:com.google.android.gms:merge_heart_minutes
Move Minutes count				derived:com.google.active_minutes:com.google.android.gms:merge_active_minutes
Calories (kcal)				derived:com.google.calories.expended:com.google.android.gms:merge_calories_expend
Distance (m)				derived:com.google.distance.delta:com.google.android.gms:merge_distance_delta
Step count				derived:com.google.step_count.delta:com.google.android.gms:merge_step_deltas
Inactive duration (hrs)				Derived
Walking duration (hrs)				Derived
Sleep(Hours)				derived:com.google.sleep.segment:com.google.android.gms:merged
Min Stress(%)		Manually collected from Smart Watch		raw:com.custom.mind.stress:292824132082:custom:model1:stress2bf
Max Stress(%)				raw:com.custom.mind.stress:292824132082:custom:model1:stress2bf
Average Stress(%)				raw:com.custom.mind.stress:292824132082:custom:model1:stress2bf
Min Stress				
Avg Stress				
Max Stress	Derived			
Mind State				
Physical State				

- { "@id": "dtmi:example:Heart;1," "@type": "Interface," "displayName": "Heart," "contents": [{"@type": "Property," "name": "AverageRate," "schema": "double" }, { "@type": "Property," "name": "MinimumRate," "schema": "double" }, { "@type": "Property," "name": "MaximumRate," "schema": "double" }, { "@type": "Property," "name": "AverageBloodOxygen," "schema": "double" }, { "@type": "Property," "name": "Points," "schema": "double" }], "@context": "dtmi:dtdl:context;2" }

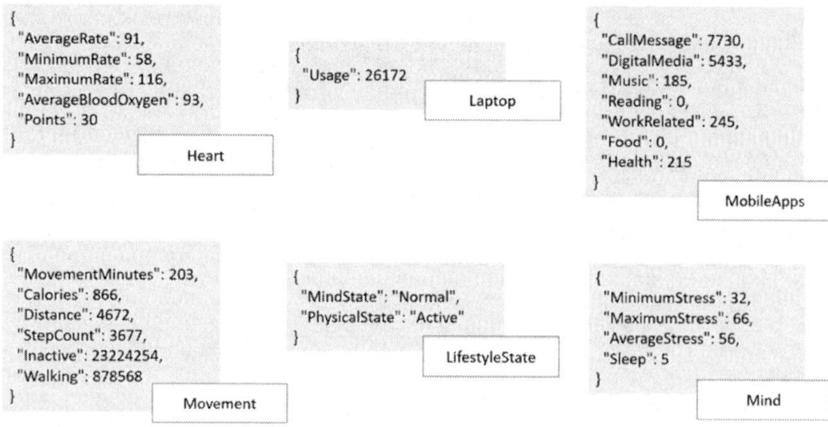

Figure 6. Dataset group for Digital Twin.

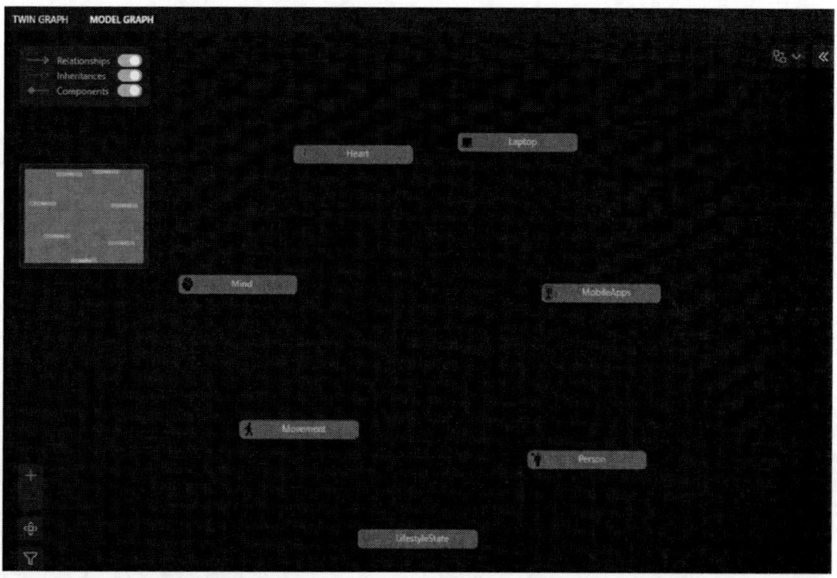

Figure 7. Digital Twin Model graph.

- In our experiment we have collected two-person health data set to simulate and predict the Lifestyle state, two twin instances of the above models are created by uploading the Twin model relationship file to Azure Digital Twin Explorer, the file will contain instances of the models and relationships between them.

Table 3 and Table 4 shows the Person 1 and Person 2 twin model and relationship respectively

- Azure Digital Twin Explorer provides an SQL-like syntax to query the Digital Twin concerning its properties, models, and relationships. The query can be submitted to Azure Digital twins using Azure Digital Twins Explorer or SDKs. Figure 8 and 9 shows the query result of Digital twins instances created on Azure.

Table 3. Twin model and relationship of Person 1

ModelID	ID (must be unique)	Relationship (From)	Relationship Name	Init Data
dtmi:example:Person;1	Person1			
dtmi:example:Laptop;1	Laptop1	Person1	contains	{"Usage": 26172}
dtmi:example:Heart;1	Heart1	Person1	contains	{"AverageRate": 91, "MinimumRate": 58, "MaximumRate": 116, "AverageBloodOxygen": 93, "Points": 30}
dtmi:example:Movement;1	Movement1	Person1	contains	{"MovementMinutes": 203, "Calories": 866, "Distance": 4672, "StepCount": 3677, "Inactive": 23224254, "Walking": 878568}
dtmi:example:Mind;1	Mind1	Person1	contains	{"MinimumStress": 32, "MaximumStress": 66, "AverageStress": 56, "Sleep": 5}
dtmi:example:MobileApps;1	MobileApps1	Person1	contains	{"CallMessage": 7730, "DigitalMedia": 5433, "Music": 185, "Reading": 0, "WorkRelated": 245, "Food": 0, "Health": 215}
dtmi:example:LifestyleState;1	LifestyleState1	Person1	contains	{"MindState":"Normal", "PhysicalState": "Active"}

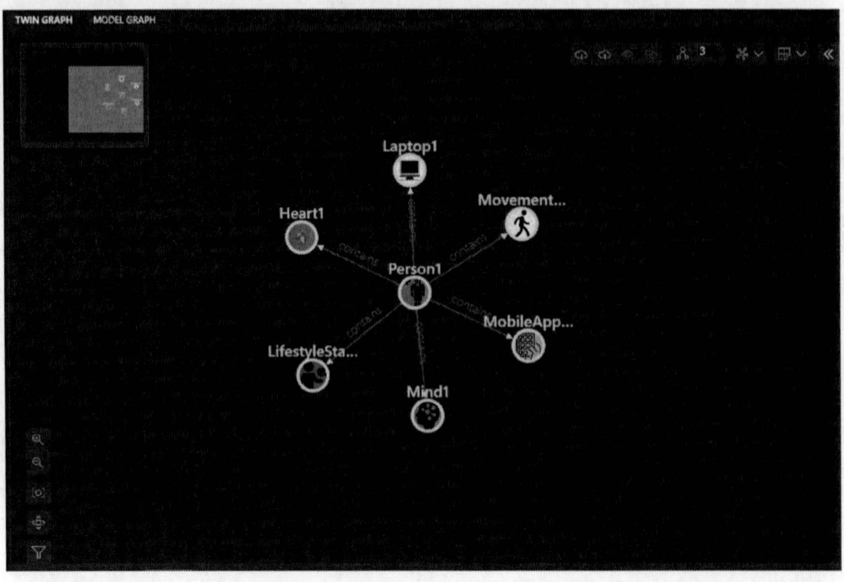

Figure 8. Digital twin instances of Person1.

2. Digital twin data update: Initial property values are provided to Azure Digital twin through the "initData" Parameter, which is a JSON string containing the relevant data. The real-time data is replaced to the Digital twin by updating multiple properties of the twin at once in JSON Patch format using the "UpdateDigitalTwin()" method. A

patch called can update as many properties on a single twin. The current twin properties and values are collected using the "GetDigitalTwin" API. The "UpdateDigitalTwin()" method can also be used to migrate a digital twin to a different model. Azure Digital Twins ensures that all incoming requests are processed sequentially to avoid any conflict.

Table 4. Twin model and relationship of Person 2

ModelID	ID (must be unique)	Relationship (From)	Relationship Name	Init Data
dtmi:example:Person;1	Person2			
dtmi:example:Laptop;1	Laptop2	Person2	contains	{"Usage": 26172}
dtmi:example:Heart;1	Heart2	Person2	contains	{"AverageRate": 91, "MinimumRate": 58, "MaximumRate": 116, "AverageBloodOxygen": 93, "Points": 30}
dtmi:example:Movement;1	Movement2	Person2	contains	{"MovementMinutes": 203, "Calories": 866, "Distance": 4672, "StepCount": 3677, "Inactive": 23224254, "Walking": 878568}
dtmi:example:Mind;1	Mind2	Person2	contains	{"MinimumStress": 32, "MaximumStress": 66, "AverageStress": 56, "Sleep": 5}
dtmi:example:MobileApps;1	MobileApps2	Person2	contains	{"CallMessage": 7730, "DigitalMedia": 5433, "Music": 185, "Reading": 0, "WorkRelated": 245, "Food": 0, "Health": 215}
dtmi:example:LifestyleState;1	LifestyleState2	Person2	contains	{"MindState":"Normal", "PhysicalState": "Active"}

3. Digital twin data analysis and Simulation: To collect, display, and analyze historical or daily data, Azure Digital Twins is integrated with Azure Time Series Insights (TSI). Azure Time Series Insights Gen2 is an end-to-end IoT analytics solution that also is scalable. It is used to collect, process, store, query, and visualize Internet of Things (IoT) data at scale. It detects hidden patterns, discovers anomalies, and does root-cause analysis. It provides Rich analytics with enhanced query APIs and user experience. Updated Digital Twin data is fed into Azure TSI through Event Hubs and Azure Function. Two event hubs and one Azure function .NET application are created to feed the incoming twin update data to Azure TSI. One event hub is used to receive twin change events, pass them to the azure function app. Azure function app converts JSON patch format to data that is highly contextualized and optimized for TSI. Another event hub is used to read the converted JSON from the Azure function and feed it into the Azure TSI. Figure 10 Shows the Architecture for the integration. Digital twin's data are stored as a flat hierarchy in Time Series Insights. Data updated into the Azure Digital Twins will flow to Azure Time Series Insight (TSI) as shown in Figure 11.

4.1. Artificial Intelligence

For AI prediction model, we have used built two model. This is a regression problem. There are two output variable, physical state and mind state. Both the variables range from 0 to 100, zero being the bad one while hundred being the best state.

Below Table gives more details for better understanding of output variables:

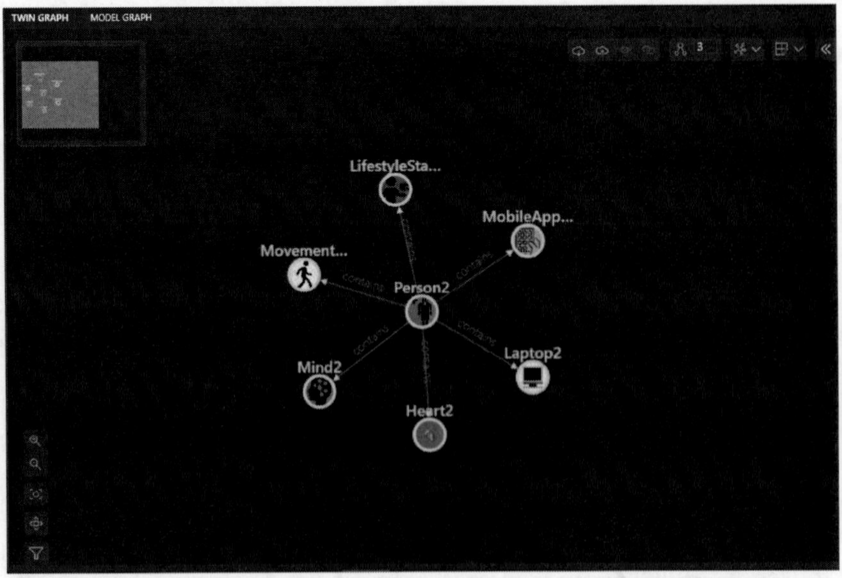

Figure 9. Digital twin instances of Person 2.

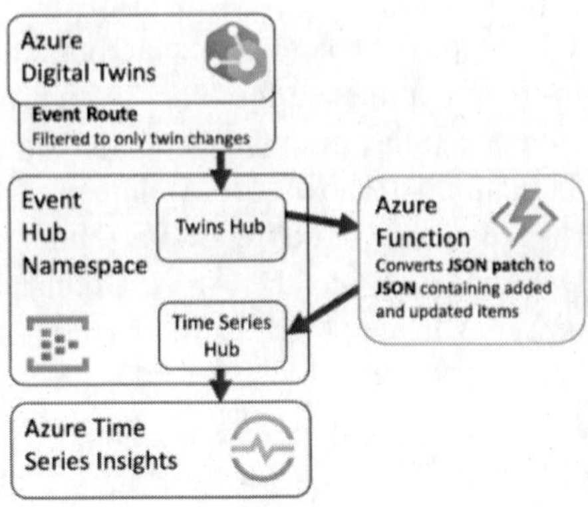

Figure 10. Source: Microsoft Azure Digital Twin and Azure TSI Integration architecture.

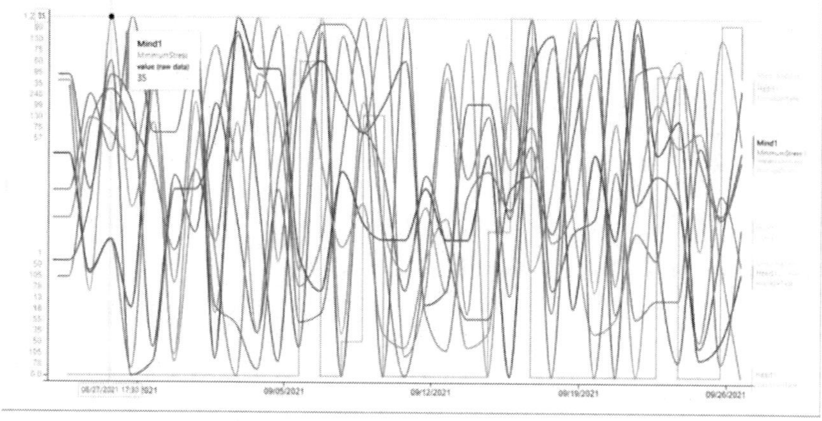

Figure 11. Azure Digital Twin Data Visualization.

Table 5. Output parameters

Mind State	Min Score	Max Score	Physical State	Min Score	Max Score
Stressed	90	100	Energized	81	100
High	80	90	Active	51	80
Medium	60	79	Normal	51	60
Normal	30	59	Lazy	31	50
Relax	0	29	Sick/Indisposed	0	30

4.1.1. AI Model

There are multiple regression models. We have tried Linear regression, logistic regression and Gradient Boosting Decision Trees (GBDT) for this problem to solve. At the end, we have finalized GBDT for our analysis.

Gradient Tree Boosting, also known as Gradient Boosted Decision Trees (GBDT), is a type of boosting that applies to any differentiable loss function. GBDT is an off-the-shelf approach that may be used to solve regression and classification problems in a wide range of applications. GB builds an additive model in a stage-by-stage manner, allowing for the optimization of any differentiable loss function. A regression tree is fitted on the negative gradient of the supplied loss function at each level.

We have built two independent models for physical and mind state. These models are built separately for each user to understand their customized nature.

For evaluation, Mean Squared Error (MSE) is considered. The mean squared error function calculates the expected value of the squared (quadratic) error or loss, which is a risk indicator.

Data was collected for nearly 6 months starting from 1st April 2021 to 12th of Oct 2021. This is further split into training and testing using Date feature.

4.2. Exploratory Data Analysis

6 months data points are collected for two users for the analysis.

1. Mobile Screen usage –

Table 6. Raw data snapshot

App name	Date	Time	Duration
App Usage	25-09-2021	11:34:46 AM	00:00:01
WhatsApp	25-09-2021	11:34:43 AM	00:00:03
Office	25-09-2021	11:34:00 AM	00:00:43
WhatsApp	25-09-2021	11:33:51 AM	00:00:09
App Usage	25-09-2021	11:32:05 AM	00:01:39
WhatsApp	25-09-2021	11:30:45 AM	00:01:03
Dainik Bhaskar	25-09-2021	11:29:57 AM	00:00:47
WhatsApp	25-09-2021	11:27:50 AM	00:02:07
YouTube	25-09-2021	11:27:26 AM	00:00:02
Screen on (unlocked)	25-09-2021	11:27:26 AM	00:00:00
Screen on (locked)	25-09-2021	11:27:26 AM	00:00:01
Screen off	25-09-2021	11:06:51 AM	00:20:34
YouTube	25-09-2021	10:22:34 AM	00:44:17
Chrome	25-09-2021	10:22:32 AM	00:00:02

Table 7 displays derived data points from above raw data and divided into 7 categories:

2. Laptop usage – overall
3. Smart Watch Data –
4. Personal Details – DOB, Gender, height, weight, Job Role, working shift

Next section is the detailed understanding of person wise dataset. It is represented in statistical graphical form.

Table 7. Derived mobile usage data

Call_Message	DigitalMedia	Music	Reading	WorkRelated	Food	Health
Zoom	Instagram	Gaana	DainikBhaskar	Gmail	Swiggy	StepSetGo
Call	Facebook	WynkMusic	Google News	Outlook	Zomato	Fit
Phone	YouTube	Amazon Music	Kindle	Teams	Dominos	Home Workout
Contacts	Twitter		Inshorts			
Contacts and dialer	LinkedIn		Apple News			
Messaging	Amazon		Daily Hunt			
WhatsApp	Prime Video					
Snapchat	discovery+					
Messages	Netflix					
Telegram	Flipkart					
Messenger	ZEE5					
Messaging	Sharechat					
Duo						

Table 8. Smart Watch Data

Average heart rate (bpm)
Max heart rate (bpm)
Min heart rate (bpm)
Sleep (Hours)
Average Blood Oxygen (%)
Move Minutes count
Calories (kcal)
Distance (m)
Step count
Heart Points
Inactive duration (hr)
Walking duration (hr)
Min Stress (%)
Max Stress (%)

4.2.1. Person 1

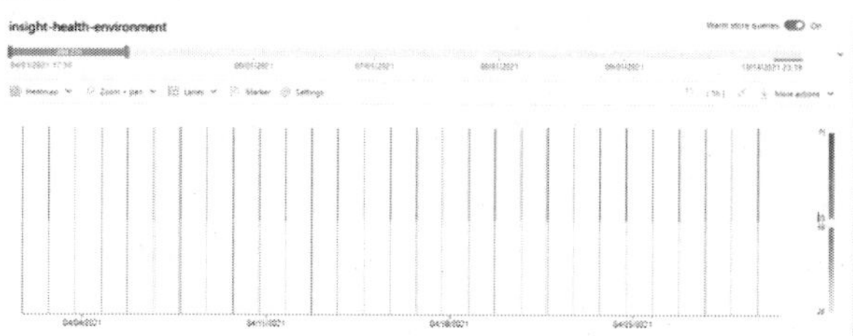

Figure 12. Heat map of Physical and Mental score of April 2021.

1. Mind State:

Below are the AI Model statistics for Mind state:

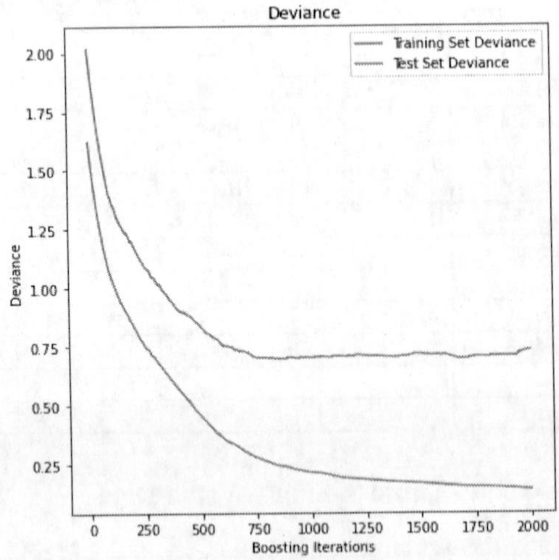

Figure 13. Training and testing dataset deviance.

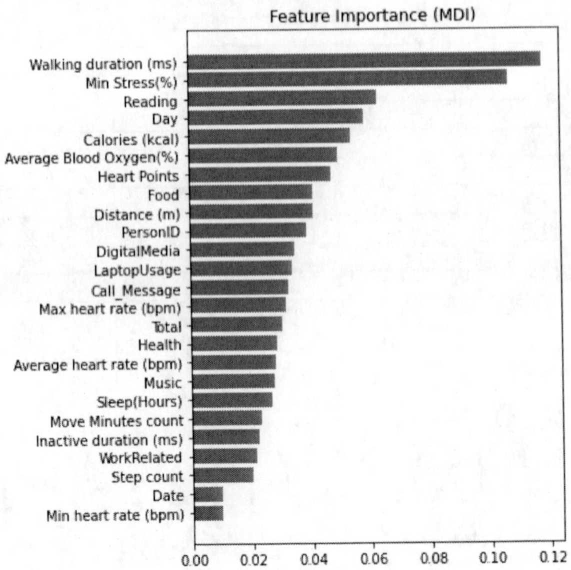

Figure 14. Feature importance of Mind state model.

- For user 1, the impurity-based and permutation techniques both reveal the same two highly predictive features: walking duration and minimum stress. It is not, however, in the same order.
- After the 1000 boosting iterations, the deviance is getting steady.

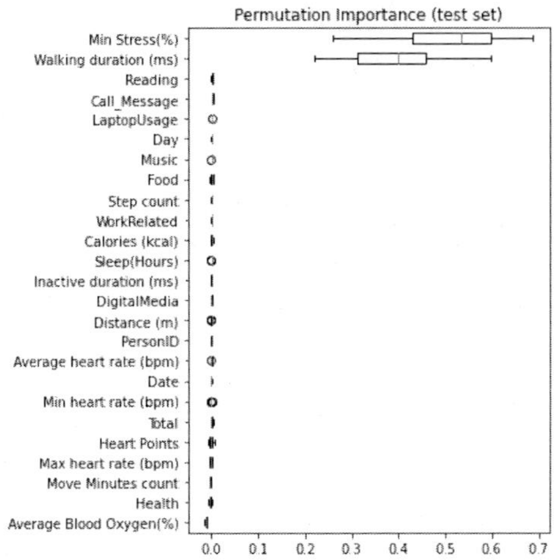

Figure 15. Permutation method representation to show feature importance.

2. Physical State

Below are the AI Model statistics for physical state:

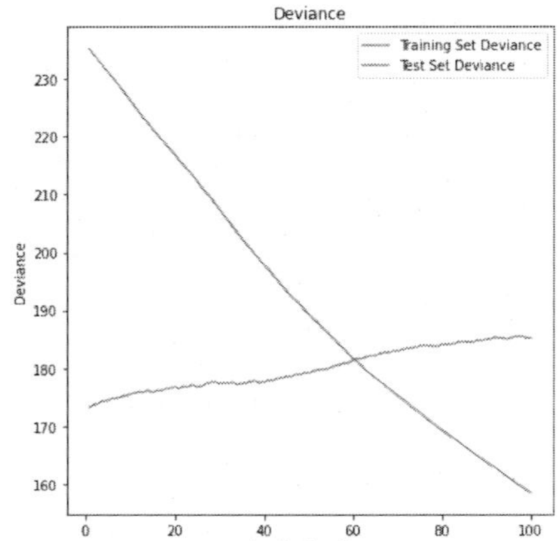

Figure 16. Training and testing dataset deviance.

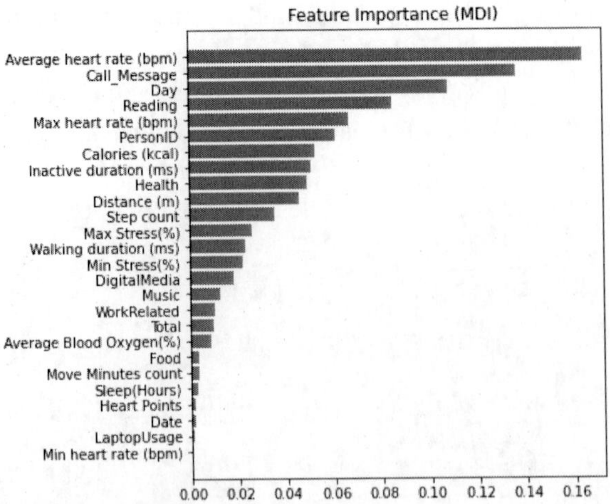

Figure 17. Feature importance of Mind state model.

4.2.2. Person 2

1. Mind state

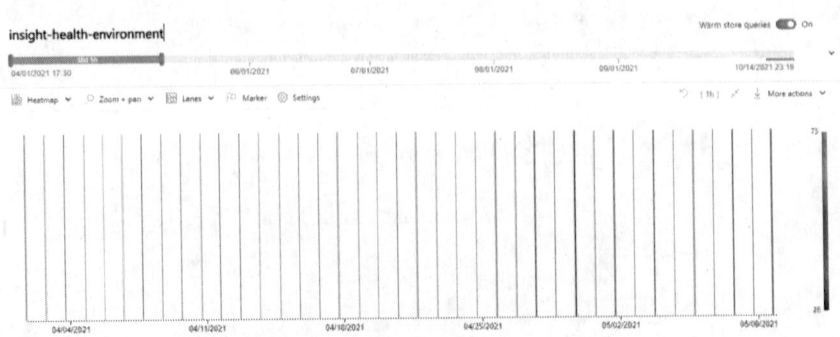

Figure 18. Mind score of Person 2 in April 2021.

Below are the AI Model statistics for Mind state:

For user 2, the impurity-based and permutation techniques uncover radically distinct predictive patterns. After the 400 boosting iterations the deviance is getting steady.

2. Physical State

Below are the AI Model statistics for physical state:

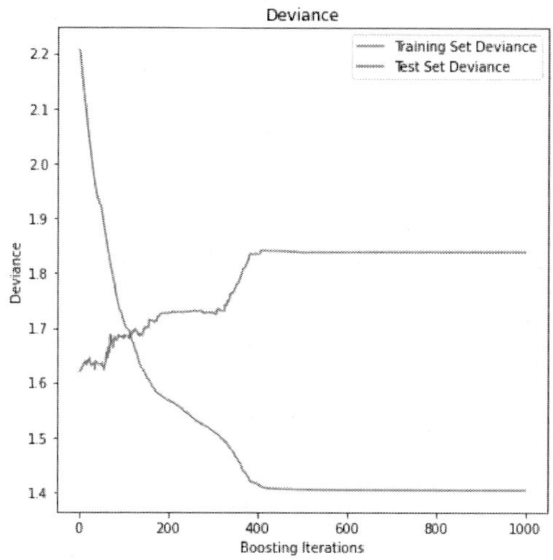

Figure 19. Training and testing dataset deviance.

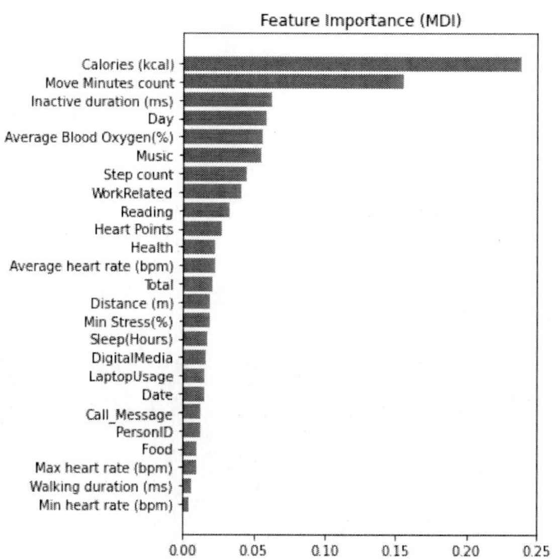

Figure 20. Feature importance of Mind state model.

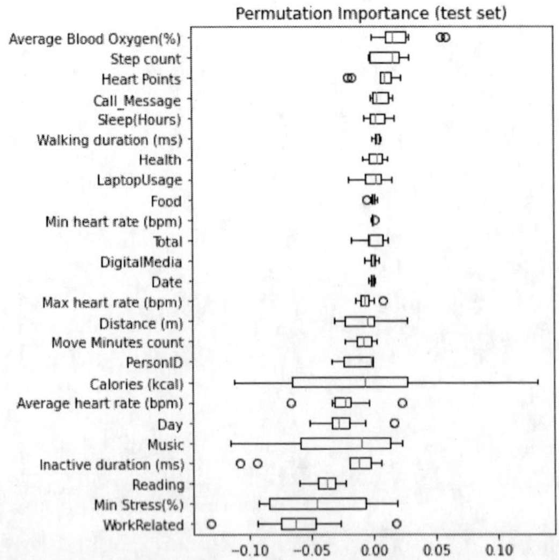

Figure 21. Permutation method representation to show feature importance.

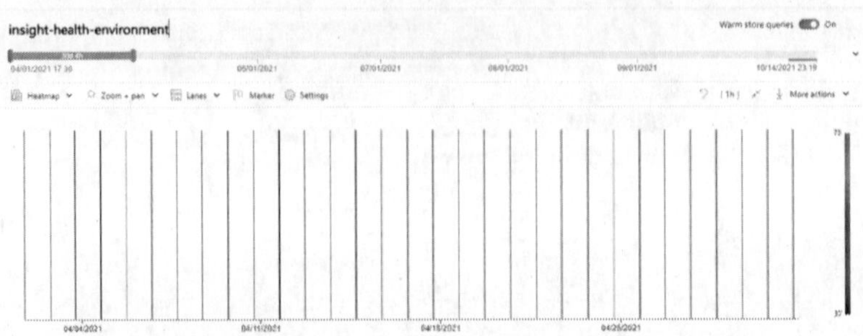

Figure 22. Physical State score in April 2021.

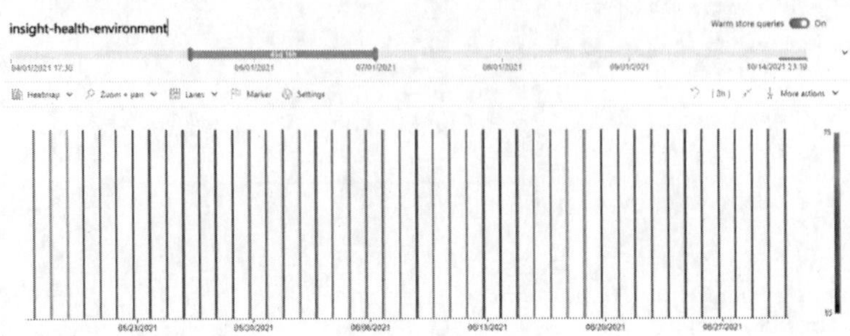

Figure 23. Physical state score in June 2021.

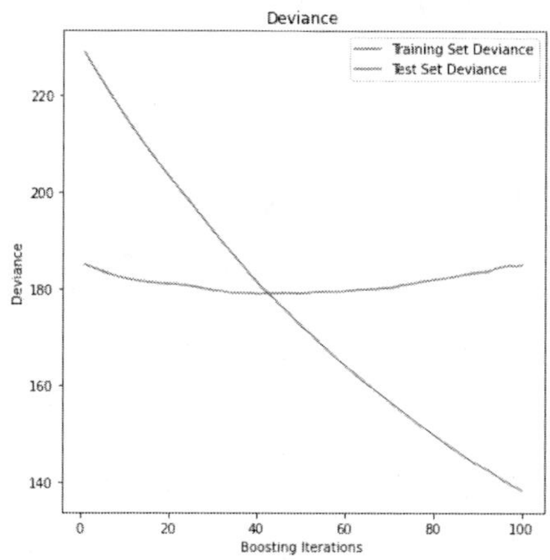

Figure 24. Training and testing dataset deviance.

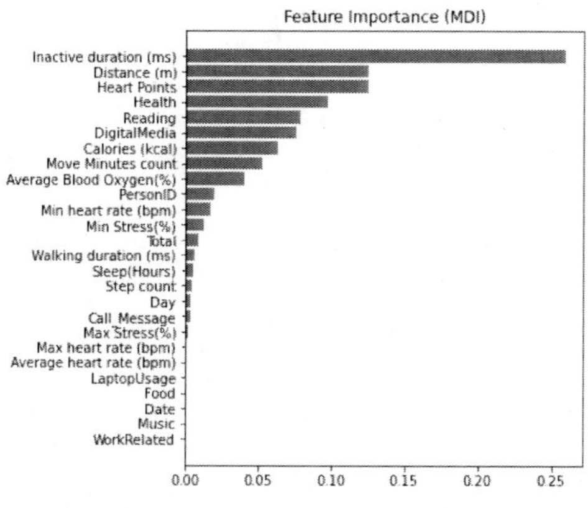

Figure 25. Feature importance of Mind state model.

4.2.3. Overall Data Analysis

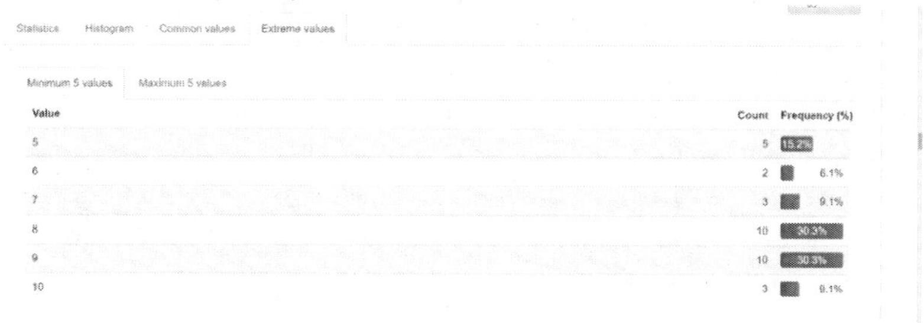

Value	Count	Frequency (%)
5	5	15.2%
6	2	6.1%
7	3	9.1%
8	10	30.3%
9	10	30.3%
10	3	9.1%

Figure 26. Sleeping hours.

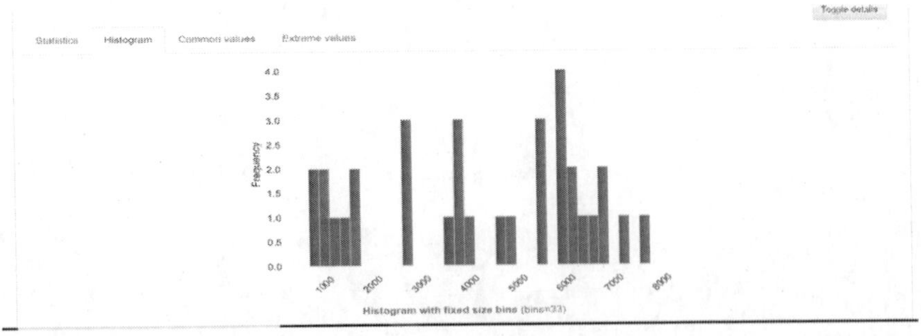

Figure 27. Time spent in seconds on Digital Media.

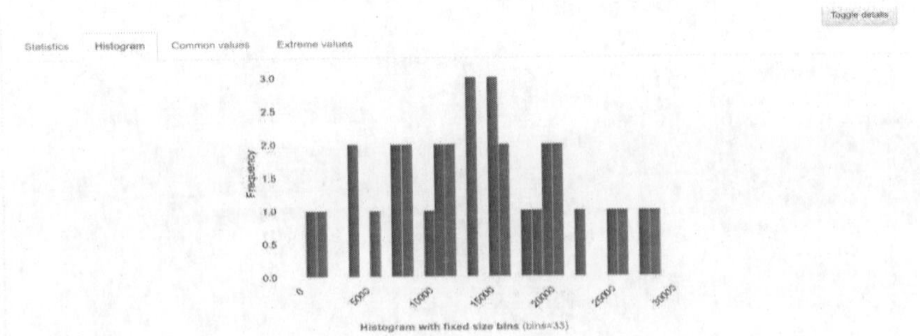

Figure 28. Time spent in seconds on calls and messages.

5. Experiment and Results Discussion

This is observed that physical state and mind state are affected by different parameters for both the users. Each individual is different, and a customized user specific model would be the best fit in this scenario.

Conclusion and Future Scope

One of the key objectives of this chapter is to understand the many data sources that influence a normal person's overall lifestyle (not having any specific severe disease). We have been successful in identifying those parameters and thorough understanding of their effects on lifestyle. Also, we have successfully integrated all the parameters into one system and provided a visualization in form of Azure TSI. The main challenge here was getting the actual data. We finally narrowed down our problem to 2 specific users from our team only and collected the original data.

Table 9. Model metrics

User 1			User 2	
Mind State	Physical State		Mind State	Physical State
0.9	.63	Train MSE	.81	.39
0.53	.24	Test MSE	.84	.21
Walking duration, minimum stress, Reading	Average heart rate, Call_Messages, Day, Reading	Important Features	Calories, Move minutes, Inactive duration	Inactive duration, distance. Heart points
{'n_estimators': 2000, 'max_depth': 10, 'min_samples_split': 2, 'learning_rate': 0.01, 'loss': 'quantile'}	{'n_estimators': 5000, 'max_depth': 10, 'min_samples_split': 2, 'learning_rate': 0.01, 'loss': 'quantile'}	Hyper parameters	{'n_estimators': 1000, 'learning_rate': 0.02, 'loss': 'quantile'}	{'n_estimators': 100, 'learning_rate':0.008, 'alpha': .8}

Collecting more data from many users and constructing the first level of a generic model to predict lifestyle states for different age groups is one of the primary objectives that should be included in future work. This will help build customized applications for individuals. Implement 3D Digital twin modelling and simulation for better user experience.

Furthermore, by integrating more data points related to medical issues, we plan to extend this work to assist medical professionals in providing better care to their patients.

References

https://databrowser.researchallofus.org/fitbit.

https://economictimes.indiatimes.com/tech/tech-bytes/fitness-and-meditation-apps-see-increased-usage-as-indians-ease-out-stress/articleshow/82320594.cms.

https://play.google.com/store/apps/details?id=com.a0soft.gphone.uninstaller.

https://ruralindiaonline.org/en/library/resource/national-mental-health-survey-of-india-2015-16-summary/.

https://swachhindia.ndtv.com/world-mental-health-day-2020-in-numbers-the-burden-of-mental-disorders-in-india-51627/.

https://takeout.google.com/?pli=1.

https://www.statista.com/statistics/558610/number-of-mobile-internet-user-in-india/.

https://www.who.int/news-room/q-a-detail/determinants-of-health.

Chapter 9

Explainable Artificial Intelligence in Smart Health Care Systems

Tawseef Ayoub Shaikh[1,*], Tabasum Rasool[1,†] and Abrar Rasool[2,‡]

[1]Department of Computer Science & Engineering, Pandit Deen Dayal Energy University, Gujrat, India
[2]Interdiciplanry Center for Water Research Indian Institute of Science, Bangalore, India
[3]Department of Electrical Engineering, Vellore Institute of Technology, Vellore, Chennai, India

Abstract

Introduction: With recent breakthroughs in organized and amorphous data and rapid growth in analysis methodologies, Artificial Intelligence (AI) is causing a revolution in the health care industry. The value of Artificial Intelligence in health care is becoming recognized at the same time that people are becoming concerned about the models' possible lack of explainability and bias. This discusses the concept of explainable artificial intelligence (XAI), which enhances a system's trustworthiness, resulting in more widespread AI adoption in health care. In this chapter, we discuss several perspectives on explainable artificial intelligence principles, as well as the understandability and interpretability of explainable AI systems, with a particular focus on the health care sector. This chapter uses AI explainability as a way to help build trustworthiness

*Corresponding Author's Email: Tawseef.Shaikh@pdpu.ac.in.
†Corresponding Author's Email: tabasumr@iisc.ac.in.
‡Corresponding Author's Email: abrardarmuntazir@gmail.com.

In: AI-Enabled IoT for Smart Health Care Systems
Editors: Tawseef Ayoub Shaikh, Tabasum Rasool and Mohammed Wasid
ISBN: 978-1-68507-977-2

in the medical domain and takes a look at the recent developments in the area of explainable AI, which encourages creativity and at times are necessary in practice to raise awareness. The goal is to teach health care providers about the interpretability and understandability of explainable AI systems.

Keywords: explainable artificial intelligence, smart health care system, black box, deep learning, machine learning

1. Introduction

The capabilities of modern machine learning-based AI systems are extensive, particularly in visual tasks [1], strategic games [2], as well as cell phone cameras that identify and track faces [3], and online services that can analyse and translate written texts [4]. In addition, artificial intelligence and machine learning have become an indispensable part of the sciences for such things as simulation and exploration [5]. Many impressive accomplishments by AI systems are due to deep learning perfections [6], plenty of big data sets being available [7], and a good amount of computational resources [8]. Advances in statistical machine learning brought AI medical research to the point where the capabilities had surpassed human performance by 1997. In the historic Lee Sedol (a top Go player) vs. DeepMind (an artificial intelligence system built by DeepMind) GO match, the 37th move demonstrated the immutability of artificial intelligence and highlighted the wealth of knowledge that might be found. AlphaGo made an unexpected move in this game, which was commented on by a Go expert in the following way. It is not a human move. I've never seen a human play this move" (Fan Hui, 2016). The same move, alternatively, was the deciding move for AlphaGo to win the game [9]. However, AlphaGo's move helped decide the game in the end. AlphaGo did not provide an explanation but rather indicated that its subsequent move revealed its intentions. In this instance, the inability to understand and test AlphaGo's decision process was not an issue, but in many cases, it may be necessary. It would be foolish to trust predictions of black-box systems, for example, medical diagnosis.

Even with this fantastic capability, obstacles remain that slow or even impede the incorporation of AI in all areas of business. The greatest challenge of deep learning models is their complexity and high demand for energy [10], which inhibits deployment in resource-constrained environments, their susceptibility to adversarial attack, and explains that trustworthiness [11], and their lack of clarity, that build a serious security hazard in applications like autonomous vehicles [12]. Currently available AI models fall short in their ability to be described or understood by clinicians due to the complexity of black-box techniques. In order for AI models to be used in medical practice in general, it is critical for both accuracy and transparency and for those making the predictions to have the ability to explain the results of the models. There is an urgent need for clinicians to understand the models' cognitive workings in order to gain trust in their predictions and find cases in which the model's predictions are flawed. In other words, an explanation need to incorporate the relevant aspects of an AI model while also conveying the clinician's causal expectations to make it valuable. The harder we try to make a visible explanation, the less meaningful it is.

Examples of automated computerised models explain to users with a good understanding of the topics like the source of the prediction [13], explanation that is incomprehensible representations. XAI offers creative ideas to back up the prediction made by any automated system. Is it always necessary to give explanations in health care? Fairness is what is most important. There are no places for humans to hide when machine learning models are involved [14]. The prognoses of these forecasts can impact the course of the patient's life greatly: diagnoses, performing surgery, or sending a patient to a hospice and a mistake costing very high costs. Misdiagnosis of a cancerous tumour can be detrimental when an unexpected theory is propounded. Pneumonia patients with asthma had a lower risk of dying [15]. When a new/unknown hypothesis is drawn, legitimisation is required as it is a critical right to information. Predictive methods alone do not guarantee results. The problem with these successful models, however, is that they usually apply in a black-box manner; that is, they don't provide any information as to how they arrive at their conclusions. Increasingly developed means for visualising, communicating, and interpreting deep learning in medical applications have newly earned much of devotion. Figure 1 demonstrates the working of traditional AI systems and an XAI system.

Still, correlation is not causation, and effective models are often black boxes. It's important to continue developing algorithms that can be explained. The explainable AI (XAI) demands to develop methods which will indicate what variables are important for results; like in the medical domain, there is a necessity for causability: We define causability as measuring the probability that any given explanation has a particular outcome; quality as measuring the strength of impact. In the future, we will continue to define human-AI relationships with explanations, as well as "what-if" scenarios, for which explainability and causability contribute a pivotal role. Medical causability is a crucial consideration because multiple factors may influence a result. Our advances in machine learning will also lead to understanding innovative designs and policies in fields like drug development and material science. The explanations will enable us to comprehend why the system arrived at the conclusions, such as, for example, in classifying patients and linking properties to new medications. There are numerous future research opportunities that are opened up by this discovery.

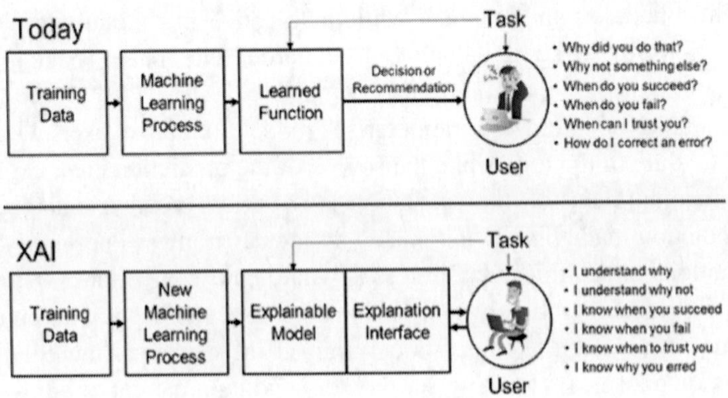

Figure 1. Traditional vs. Explainable Artificial Intelligence.

To make machine learning models, we acknowledge two varieties of models: Black-box and the Glass-box.

i. Black-box models: It is typical for most black-box models to have a great deal of dissonance, as there is no way to know how it was arrived at the solution in the first place and provide poor interpretability; thus, tradeoffs must be made. Several model-agnostic methods are used to initialise black box models. A characteristic of most ML algorithms due to the fact that domain experts are unable to decipher the algorithm's mathematical processes. Since machine learning models aren't transparent about their inner workings, these approaches are applied to better understand the output that occurs during the black box phase of machine learning [16].

ii. Glass-box models: Imply that all necessary information is readily available, tradeoff for such a method is often the models' performance for an explainable solution; the term glass-box can often be thought of as synonymous with the term XAI. Glass-box methods have seen recent implementation with the likes of models such as the Explainable Boosting Machine (EBM) and DeepLIFT. EBM is a glass-box model introduced by Microsoft in 2019 [17]. The architecture of DeepLIFT can be used in junction with model agnostic methods such as SHAP (Shapley Additive exPlanations), an explanatory method; this can be seen in the DeepSHAP implementation and their various hybridisations [18].

1.1. Explainable Artificial Intelligence (XAI)

Van lent et al. [19], 2004, introduced the term to the definition of AI-controlled entities in computer games in their research paper of that year. In layman's terms, AI is basically explainable, but no generally accepted standard exists for explainable AI. According to DARPA [20], XAI's goals are to "produce more explainable models while maintaining a high level of learning performance (prediction accuracy) and enable human users to understand, appropriately, trust, and effectively manage the emerging generation of artificially intelligent partners". The goal of enable ability in fat-friendly analytics, as stated by the FAT [21], is toensure that algorithmic decisions, as well as any data driving those decisions, can be explained to end-users and other stakeholders in non-technical terms". FICO [22], the sponsor of the XML Challenge, sees it as "an innovation towards opening up the black-box of ML" and as a challenge to create models and techniques that are both accurate and provide a good trustworthy explanation that will satisfy customers' needs". Figure 2 describes the commonly used interchangeable synonyms words of XAI in the literature.

Most projects utilising XAI concentrate in the ultra-critical scenarios, including automated transportation, intelligent health care, defence, and financial sectors.

1.1.1. Automated Transportation

It holds the promise of lessening the number of traffic deaths because of self-driving vehicles while also challenging the explainability of AI decisions. Decisions made by self-driving vehicles must be made instantaneously based on objects in the view of the camera. When an autonomous vehicle does something other than what it is programmed to do, the outcome can be devastating. This has already occurred back in late March when a self-driving Uber vehicle struck and killed a pedestrian in Tempe, Arizona. The first reported fatality that involved a totally self-driving vehicle. The object that was located in front of the vehicle was reported by unidentified individuals, who alleged the software incorrectly identified it as a tumbleweed or a plastic bag [23]. Only a clear explanation will explain these ambiguous circumstances if they ever arise.

Figure 2. XAI Word Cloud.

1.1.2. Smart Health Care Systems

The medical model determines who lives and who dies. We'll never be able to treat a patient as directed by a black box unless we've validated the diagnosis. Artificial neural networks learned to provide clinical decisions in the mid-1990s: Results showed that an ANN could predict which patients needed to be admitted to the hospital and which could be treated there. Neural nets were found to be significantly more accurate than classical approaches at first, but subsequent results contradicted the findings. Nevertheless, after much testing, it was found that the neural network inferred that people with pneumonia had a lower risk of death and didn't require hospitalisation. Medically, this is contrary to our previous assumption, but these patients with pneumonia were more likely to be admitted to the ICU than, to begin with, and this treatment demonstrated an obvious clinical pattern in the training data. In conclusion, it was then decided to discontinue the AI program since it was more likely to harm than help [24]. We must interpret the model if we want to avoid this critical design problem.

1.1.3. Legal

AI could reduce both crime and criminal re-recidivism costs in the criminal justice system. However, when it comes to the risk of recidivism in criminal decisions, we must make sure that the formula is neutral, fair, and not discriminatory. Mr. Loomis was convicted of having used proprietary, closed source sentencing software in Loomis v. Wisconsin case [25]. A process right was violated when the software COMPAS (Correctional Offender Management and Program Placement for Alternative Sanction), took race and gender into consideration [26]. As the algorithm was a trade secret, the judge was unaware of the causal steps involved in the process.

1.1.4. Finance

Advances in capital administration, admittance to investment advice and service, and greater value for customers are all brought about by the use of artificial intelligence. It should be noted, however, that these solutions create issues around data security and fair lending as well. As you know, loan 'underwriters' inducers are strictly regulated and are legally obligated to make sound decisions. Another challenge of employing AI-based models in the scoring and lending process is that the reasons behind the denial of credit must be coded in detail. Even when the source of the denial is an unknown ML algorithm, there may be validity in the claim.

1.1.5. Military

Until recently, XAI was the brainchild of military researchers and has grown in popularity thanks to DAPRA calls for additional research. The complexities of depend on self-governing systems for military operations are examined in a study from MIT Technology Review [27, 28].

1.2. Background

Various solutions of XAI have been proposed over the years in the health care domain, many of which have been put into practice. When it comes to the use of XAI, some algorithms can be completely explained by their design, such as the analysis of medical conditions via an IF-THEN process (asthma, diabetes, lung cancer) that also allows researchers to explain the diagnosis (and sometimes the prediction of the disease) using their medical record profile [29]. Let's take, for example, a condition such as "the patient is a smoker and has a respiratory illness" and use it to predict if lung cancer will occur. It's tricky to explain what comes first, the horse or the cart: however, the challenge with self-explanatory models is that they limit the uses of others to increase the accuracy of their own predictions. Because of a surge in generalisable AI models, the use of extensible AI models has grown to meet this demand [30]. They are also known as model-agnostic XAI methods because their applications are not connected to the model that needs to be explained [30]. Using a commonly used model-agnostic approach, Local Interpretable Model-Agnostic Explanation (LIME), researchers [31] tried to explain their predictions by identifying all of the interacting variables. These researchers [32] used LIME to show that Recurrent Neural Networks (RNNs) are useful in identifying conditions such as kidney failure, anemia, and diabetes that increase the risk of heart failure. In addition, various other XAI models have been used for model agnostic techniques in the health care domain, such as anchors, Shapley values [34, 34]. As in [35], a design framework proposes to make better explanations by harnessing the knowledge of human reasoning utilising user goals to develop XAI methods. Additionally, it can be applied to generate human-friendly explanations of AI-based systems throughout the entire process, helping with patient decision-making at various stages.

V. Sharma et al. [36] created an explainable AI-based prediction approach for COVID-19 risk using a two-step methodology. In combination with advanced CCT scans, the initial risk outcome analysis uses deep learning-based analytics to yield an accurate prediction of COVID-19 infection. Cost and time are minimal since this new AI perspective framework will benefit a majority of the low-income population that lacks access to advanced health care facilities. J.A. Duell et al. [37] sought to apply explainable XAI to demonstrate the ease of applying a tertiary black box model. The models used are logistic regression and Extreme Gradient Boost, which are described as black-box models. The given models are evaluated against glass box strategy and Explainable Boosting Machine like Shapley Additive exPlanations (SHAP), Local Interpretable Modelagnostic Explanations (LIME), and Scoped Rules. Two of the feature-agnostic solutions display moderate errors in their prioritisation, which finally agree on a low level of importance for all three of them. The authors [38] et al. suggested a new Explainable AI approach in health care involving two components: explanation characteristics and human-machine trust.

The authors [39] et al. backed a solution empowering the explainability of ML models and the fundamental roadmaps to be unified into the typical ML models. D. David et al. [40] examined examples from the data of the UCI, evaluating various ways of applying XAI techniques, as well as relevant use cases for it. The study in [41] described how useful explainability is for medical use and a wide variety of possible computer-aided diagnosis (CAD) applications by applying it to technological, legal, medical, and patient contexts. Artificially interpretable models can be described as the aforementioned method for predicting the risk of pneumonia [41] and rules which are constructed through generative models derived from sparse probabilistic inference [42]. However, models will generally be biased this way in order to prevent predictability in order to be interpretable [43].

Yang et al. [44] projected a recursive partitioning (GIRP) to formulate a wide variety of models based on their narrower explanations grounded on their local mechanisms. They demonstrated their methodology to identify a reasonable or unreasonable ML algorithm in practice. Ribeiro et al. [45] come up with a LIME model that is able to approximate the target locally within a prediction of any specific target class. Extended decision rules called anchors are designed and put foreword in [46]. Similarly, the leave-one covariate-out (LOCO) [47] technique is an effective way of generating local explanations. Another effort is attempted by Bahr et al. [48] for producing local explanations.

The authors in [49] et al. explained one instance by comparing the initial prediction to the univariate version. Lately, there have been many applications that use decomposition to clarify locally [50]. Bastani et al. [51] used a simulated decision tree behaviour with a surrogate model. Thiagar et al. [52] offer an alternative to using a surrogate model for TreeViewvisualizations. Tan et al. [53] experimented with model distillation to see if they could use it to separate complex models into more basic ones in an interpretable phenotype approach. Che et al. [54] introduced a new prototype known as Interpretable Mimic Learning (IML), which is used to take advantage of both traditional and deep learning models. Xu et al. [55] recently introduced a method known as DarkSight for data visualisation inspired by dark knowledge classifiers. Wachen et al. [56] presented an original concept for automated decisions called unconditional counterfactual explanations.

To learn the most similar prototypes and complaints about a given dataset, Kim et al. developed a maximum mean discrepancy (MMD) measure of similarity. Deletion diagnostics has been employed by Cook [58] et al. et al. to estimate the influence of an instance on model predictions was created to do so. The authors in [59] came up with Guided Grad-CAM in order to extract complementary heatmaps for the classification of Alzheimer's disease. DeepLight (which outputs a heatmap) is used to generate fMRI data for Human Connectome Project [60]. Gain saliency map is calculated by the gradient of loss and supplied interpretability to the neural network for EEG classification [61]. It's been noted that features within CNN are likened to skin lesions, specifically [62]. Similarly, the stroke prediction model is created from the class of Bayesian Rules in [63]. An LSTM-based mass classifier (text justification) lies in the work of [64]. In the studies in [65], a logistic regression model discovered a correlation between the likelihood of getting pneumonia and having a lower risk of dying. Getting pneumonia has a negative impact on mortality was shown to be riskier in a regression study [65]. Ridge regression is applied to the AD and schizophrenia dataset [66]. The research also offers summaries of foundational knowledge on deep learning as well as taxonomy and classifying them into taxonomy [67]. A lot of surveys contain topics relating to trend information in XAI, and show the future research directions that could be viewed in [68-71].

The purpose of this chapter is to show how to use explainable artificial intelligence (XAI) to demonstrate the usability and explainability of the commonly found machine learning black box models. The features that indicate the relative importance of a model's predictions are governed by the major concepts of XAI. Also, due to the availability of XAI, we are able to extract useful domain-related knowledge from high-dimensional data sources in order to help human decision-makers track changes, which is made possible by combining categorical and numeric elements that may be impossible for a human expert to manage. This intends to help inform decisions and place as an assistant - not a substitute to a human expert, forming a tertiary layer of knowledge, where we have: the patient data, the patient data observations from a domain expert; and an explainable solution to act as the aforementioned subsidiary tertiary layer.

The chapter proceeds as follows. Section 2 of the report looks at the importance of trust and transparency in AI. It focuses on the various attributes of the XAI in the biomedical sphere. The differences between types of explanations and the quantity of information associated with them are discussed in Section 3. The recent approaches are also explained here, including surrogate functions, frame explanation as an optimisation problem, and model explanation. Section 4 attempts to examine the quality of answers to this question. At the end of the chapter, there is a discussion of explaining XAI's general challenges and future directions in Section 5.

2. Transparency and Trust of AI in Biomedical Domain: Needs and Challenges

Although the modern sophisticated and automated machines do often outperform human experts but the question of robustness and reliability viz, how can we assure the AI solution is trustworthy, still haunts the machine learning experts. Trust is critical to machine learning in medicine, as it is required to tackle the concern of human subject treatment for machine-person modeling, and central to the machine-person scenario when held by external parties, such as insurance companies [72], like in clinical and operational settings. Human trust plays a pivotal role in human-AI collaboration ranging from the medical field to vehicle automation [73]. As the automation in various human segments gets idealises, so are the questions posed to human response and acceptance. With the intent to provide a better performing solution than a human expert alone, a commonality arises in algorithm application as to where the model can exhibit different behaviours in a non-deterministic manner compromising the trust factor to where black-box models become an adversary to trust. The work in [73] et al. surrounds the question of what clinicians want." It has been identified that simply having a highly accurate machine learning model is not enough, particularly a single metric such as accuracy that to ascertain how the solution was acquired and depth that provides insight to the methodologies involved. A learning problem will have varying per-case interpretability, depending on how obscure its approaches are. A relatively small set of machine learning algorithms are well-suited to statistical modelling. Linear regression, Logistic Regression, and a Decision Tree are interpretable models, together with Naive Bayes and k-Nearest Neighbours, since all three can be considered thelocal observations.

All patients could benefit from these advances in health care-oriented artificial intelligence systems. There is uncertainty and risk for the patient in the health care environment, which necessitates creating a patient's trust. How do we enable AI systems to trust with matters of life and death? How does trust in AI systems influence people's attitude toward health care in general? A great theory that not only integrates the facts but also explains them. AI in health care is too risky to implement just yet as a significant percentage of health care providers, in general, do not have faith in artificial intelligent automated CAD devices. The study found that 30% of clinicians, respondents lack trust in AI [74]. Not only are doctors, but also 61% of UK residents are uninterested in using AI for their health care needs [75]. There are several reasons why people don't trust AI-powered health care systems like that to be explained or well understood. For health care, there are many opportunities. Examples include assisting in diagnostic decision making, drug discovery, risk management, and patient monitoring, as well as the analysis of "big data" genomics, metabolomics, proteomics, and so on [76]. Medical imaging is relevant in pathology, radiology [77], ophthalmology [9], oncology [10], and many other medical application fields [78].

Let us examine a successful work from Stanford, which was reported in Europe in 2017 a couple of years ago as "AI is better than doctors" [79]. What on earth did they do? In this system, skin lesions were categorised using a single end-to-to-end convolution neural network (CNN) that was trained from dermal images instead of disease names, and all the classifications were done solely on pixel data. To practice image classification before the 2014 ImageNet challenge, they prepared using 1.3 million images. However, they subsequently used approximately 2,000 different clinical images and obtained a 92% average level of performance compared to dermatologists. This result is truly amazing, considering that the algorithm never gets tired. They may be satisfactory, but pressing questions are: "Why is this happening," "What variables are contributing to this," What if I decide to change, replace, distract, or remove the input data. This should consider and examine the aspects of techniques such as fidelity [80] and reproducibility [81], but also take into account other characteristics, like simplicity and generality.

A recent histopathology work from the Princess Margaret Hospital in Toronto has gone one step further [82]. Additionally, a CNN was applied to a database of 840,000 histological image tiles, and learned representation was found. This is more remarkable because it has been demonstrated that machine-generated features correlate with specific structures found in human cognition, and specifically those found in humankind. And because humans think similarly to machines, these overlaps can be important for both eliminating i) bias and ii) improving algorithms, making them more robust and understandable so that we can hold medical AI. Despite all these victories, the most important challenges remain in the computational abilities required for human-level AI, as it must be able to deal with "common sense and reason like human." To become even more useful, we need to design these approaches so they are simple, relevant, and understandable to a human expert. The design is to put the respective advantages to good use. Causality can be understood and utilised even further by medical experts.

Most importantly, note that these terms refer to methods to implement "retrospect ability, comprehensibility, and extensibility of black box" approaches. In the best practice examples we see above, these methods have delivered excellent results. Unfortunately, using black-box models for sensitive decisions means machine learning is not an option. Nevertheless, in biomedical research, there is a requirement to transcend AI. The key to comprehensible health care is an effective explanation of causation [83]. Causability encompasses quality of explanations, like heatmaps produced by AI. Artificial intelligence (AI) can be seen as an attribute that seeks to be understood, whereas causal understanding (CAI) focuses on understanding human intelligence. Understanding what it is that people expect AIs to do is a prerequisite for effective human-AI interaction and ultimately successful human-AI applications.

Black box design artificial intelligence is becoming increasingly common in today's apps. The performance of consumer electronics and online translation services is fine without complete transparency and explainability as long as the accuracy of the models is acceptable. But even if these devices fail, such as the cell phone camera, failing to identify people may be unavoidable. Transparency and trust requirements are quite minimal for these types of AI. Safety is a critical consideration in the deployment of creative and non-critical software. When it comes to less-developed methods, the uncertainty of techniques may also be a problem. As long as there is the possibility of a single incorrect decision end result leading to life or health issues or a major monetary loss, there cannot be reliance on an algorithm that cannot be understood. It is more difficult to adopt machine learning in sectors such as health, e-commerce, or entertainment because there is a greater reluctance in those areas.

2.1. "Clever Han" Predictors Explanation

This famous horse known as "Clever Hans" was able to count to calculate numbers, and people regarded him as a scientific wonder in the early part of the 20th century. Research has shown that in the vast majority of instances, Hans is able to determine the subject's mood from the reaction of the questioner. Another phenomenon has recently been noted in state-of-the-art AI systems. Additionally, here the algorithms have discovered spurious correlations in the training and test data and have likewise learned to mispredict wrong correlations in the test data. For instance, the authors of [84] showed that the PASCAL VOC competition [85] found objects not by method but by searching for correlations and the context of the data. It is able to distinguish boats and trains because of their presence in an image, and they can detect them by the presence of a watermark. The presence of copyright-related imagery in the entire horse dataset is an artefact that has long gone unnoticed by both the participants and organisers of the competition. It can be assumed that the thousands of images in the dataset have not been thoroughly searched for that type of error (but even if someone did, such artefacts might be easily overlooked). People have pointed out that there are many other examples of "Clever Hans" who did clever things. It has also been shown, for instance [86], that current deep neural networks can tell apart wolf images from husky images mainly by the fact that there is snow in the picture. The authors [87] show that smart models learn padded concepts, while academic authors [88] demonstrated that their model doesn't distinguish between dumbbells and aircraft; their model only learned to associate dumbbells with arms that lift it. Of course, "Clever Han"-type prognosticators have good predictive accuracy in the test sets but do not have good application in the real world, where horses may be found on trailers, but no "wolves" or "huskie" can be.

2.2. Explanations Foster Trust and Verifiability

It is vitally important to verify the decisions made by an AI system so people will feel confident in them (as in the medical diagnosis, for example) (e.g., autonomous driving). Explanations help the doctor to gain a holistic knowledge of the patient in order to choose the best therapy. A similar to a radiologist, who would write a report going into extensive detail explaining their findings, a support system should document their findings (e.g., doctor explaining therapy to a patient).

2.3. Characteristics/Pillars of Explainable AI in Health Care

Figure 3 below discusses the various vital pillars for Explainable AI in smart health care systems.

2.3.1. Transparency

User-friendliness of the machine learning algorithm, model, and features.

2.3.2. Domain Sense

It should be rooted in usage and acceptable to the users of the system. It could mean that the patient had a 62% chance of being readmitted in the same year as well as before, or it could mean that the patient will return 62% of the time.

2.3.3. Consistency

The theory should apply to all models and all runs of the model. Referring to the patient when you want to use his doctor is to go to see him as "left without being seen" can lead to adverse events.

2.3.4. Consistency|Model Multiplicity

Depending on the training data, multiple learning algorithms can produce similar results. Different theories should all point to the same response. More divergent interpretations of a problem or the underlying issues related to the problems.

2.3.5. Parsimony

If a clarification is necessary, it should be as short as possible. It 'shouldn't be difficult to express the complexities of the description, but has some points to make about the functionality. If a patient is admitted, the decision will reflect where they will be placed in the hospital.

2.3.6. Generalizability|Length of Stay Prediction

As long as the model can be applied to other problems, so should the description. A hospital stay is described by the length of time the patient spends there.

2.3.7. Trust/Performance

An assumption of a predictive algorithm must have a certain level of performance. Predicting the need for ICU transfer is ICU transfer prediction.

2.3.8. Fidelity

When people expect an explanation and a model to be in sync, they are both disappointed if the predictions prove incorrect. Once the patient has left the hospital, there is a good chance they will be readmitted within 30 days. Many Shadow, Surrogate, and Student models allow a clear understanding of the model's performance while avoiding error.

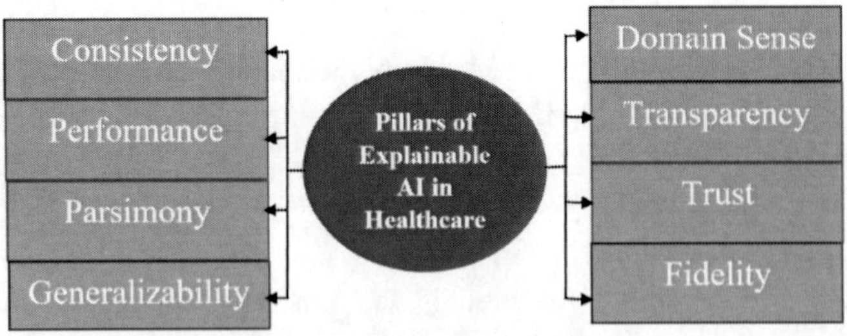

Figure 3. Characteristics of Explainable AI in Health care.

Table 1 below mentions in detail the nature of trust and transparency of various machine learning models for learning. The deep architecture of the model amplifies the black-boxing, and it becomes hard to visualise the actual working of the system. The deep learning paradigms are the main concern whose work needs to be justified by the explainable artificial intelligence (XAI), particularly when we are dealing with the biomedical domain.

Table 1. Nature of transparency of different machine learning models

Transparent	Semi-Transparent	Non-Transparent
Falling Rule Lists	Shallow Ensembles	Deep Learning
GAM (Generalised Additive Models)		SVM (Support Vector Machines)
GA2M (Generalised Additive Models with interactions)		Gradient Boosting Models
LIME (Locally Interpretable Model Agnostic Explanations)		
Naïve Bayes		
Regression Models		
Shapley Values		

3. Explanations of AI Methods in Biomedical Domain

Prevalent approaches for explaining predictions are discussed in this section.

3.1. Explaining with Surrogates (Feature-Based Techniques)

Explaining with Surrogates (feature-based techniques), traditional classifiers such as the linear model or a shallow decision tree are by default explanatory as far as their interpretability is concerned, and explaining its predictions is a triviality. Deep neural networks, in contrast, use many layers of transformations that significantly complicate classification and prediction tasks. A way to clarify the predictions of complex models is to think of, and model the phenomenon implementing them as simple approximations and Local Interpretable Model-agnostic Explanations (LIME) is one example which fits well in this domain [89]. Here, neural network is estimated in the range of interest, where it approaches the relevant input function and computes the surrogate function by finding a local maximum of the function at those points. LIME can convey a lot of information if the input domain of the surrogate function is human-readable since it is fully general. It can be used to classify any kind of model, regardless of the classifier's internal architecture, such as a GoogleNet, wherein computation, takes several minutes to be processed [90]. Comparable to LIME, SmoothGrad uses a simple neighbourhood of the input to obtain the gradient. Another excellent feature of SmoothGrad [91] is that it does not use the internals of the model; however, it does make use of the gradient. A model with the technique of Shapley Additive exPlanations (SHAP) [92] is easier to recognise and amplifies the transparency of the method for the usefulness of the concept. SHAP assigns a relative model value (comparative influence of every feature to the target aberration) and then identifies the mean prediction (the base value). The overall explanation can also be seen as both specific and global, as well as regional.

3.2. Explaining with Local Perturbations

Another class of methods analyses the model's response to the current conditions. This includes gradient and perturbation-based approaches, to information use. Explaining techniques utilising the variation of the function of interest in machine learning have a long history [93]. The second notable technique is referred to as the "Sensitivity Analysis (SA""[94]. Although widely applied, it actually provides an explanation rather than merely describing the change. Furthermore, SA is found to be fundamentally flawed because of gradient discontinuities and gradient shattering, and explanation discontinuity issues, which is often cited as being suboptimal for modern AI models [95]. Perturbation methods clearly test the model's rejoinder to more general local perturbations [96]. While the occlusion method [97] gauges the importance of input dimensions by obliterating parts of the input, the Prediction Difference Analysis (PDA) [98] analyses an individual feature pixel by pixel and yields true information. An issue for all model-agnostic approaches, such as neural networks, is that they have to be retrained to consider every possible perturbation [99]. Sometimes other methods employ a formulation for an explanation of the idea that constitutes an optimization problem [100].

3.3. Sensitivity Analysis

As explained by the model's locally derived partial derivative, this predicted a gradient (partial derivative) calculation briefly taking on added importance due to quantification of the relative importance of each input [101]:

$$R_i = \| \frac{\partial}{\partial x_i} f(x) \| \qquad (1)$$

This evaluation strategy assumes that the most important input characteristics are those which are most important to which output is most sensitive [101]. Sensitivity analysis does not describe the function itself but rather describes a way to analyse a variation of the function. The resulting heatmap shows which data values need to be modified to make the appearance of the system (as it sees them) more/less accurate.

3.4. Propagation-Based Approaches (Leveraging Structure)

These methods of explanation do not ignore the model they are incorporating. Layer-wise Relevance Propagation (LRP) [102] is applicable to neural networks with layers, such as LSTM [103], as well as Fisher Vector classifiers [104]. In LRP, one attempts to create a unique picture of decisions by taking the prediction of the output and redistributing it throughout the model. LRP was further modified for anomaly models like clustering and anomaly detection in recent years. The proper theoretically motivated structure of the model, along with appropriate propagation rules, yield optimal explanations at little cost of computation (one forward and one backward pass). Since LRP does not use gradients, there are no gradient issues or gradient breakage. Deconvolution [105] and Guided Backpropagation [106] are further extensions that utilises the model's internal structure. Some of these methods use heuristics; others have a pre-distribution step embedded in them.

3.5. Layer-Wise Relevance Propagation

Among the most popular forms of AI models disintegrating predictions of modern AI systems includes long-short term memory (LSTM) networks [107] and Fisher vectors [108]. In contrast to other methods of sensitivity analysis, this method identifies pivotal variables. Work published in recent years [109] also includes a decomposition analysis, which is a well-known function in mathematics. A recent classification technique called layer-wise relevance propagation (LRP) can now serve as an explanation for the classifier's decisions. Local redistribution discretization is used to calculate *f(x)* backwards, but keeps score *Ri* for each input based on importance so that importance is reflected (e.g., image pixel). With regard to relevance conservation, this redistribution process can be defined like this:

$$\sum_i R_i = \ldots = \sum_j R_j = \sum_k R_k = \ldots = f(x) \qquad (2)$$

Thus, according to this property, the total amount of relevancy (or the prediction), is always the same across the entirety of a deep neural network [109]. Redistribution does not artificially inflate or deflate relevance. The contribution score *Ri* of each input decides how significant the relevance is rather than simply weights for the *f(x)*.

3.6. Example-Based Techniques

Anchors are important to be present when a feature has a high relative relevancePrediction [110]. Here, the features are tapered down to convinced conditions (i.e., anchors), which gives the prediction. The algorithm is an extension of a model-agnostic approach to image, text, and tabular models. It's based on the If-Then algorithm, which gives it flexibility and increases the certainty of finding future instances.

3.7. Counterfactuals

Additionally, as machine learning models are applied to real-world data, we must also know "which feature should be modified in order to switch the prediction." A model-agnostic xAI approach that searches for the smallest changes to features that are possible in order to yield a different result comes under the umbrella of Counterfactual [111]. These best explain the black-box models and work optimal on binary datasets. Recursive explanations yield the best results on binary datasets. Since we can store more than two values per label in a binary classification dataset, the performance isn't as great.

3.8. Counterfactuals with Prototypes

It refers to the generic description instances, i.e., a prototype. There are several prototypes that can be used for counterfactuals, which include counterfactuals in addition to factual models [112]. According to the counterfactual method, counter-intuitive representations will work with black box models. This technique is applicable to any method of applying prototypes to your variables and is thus faster than using counter-examples. Using a prototype search technique speeds up the search time greatly because it takes the counterfactual (what you would normally be looking for) and leads it to the prototype of a particular class.

3.9. Contrastive Explanation Methods

It provides a localised explanation for a black box method. These components are not valuable for the model's classification, namely Pertinent negatives (PN) or Pertinent positives (PP). It specifies what information must be present in the model in order to retain the prediction class and the minimum information that must be provided for a meaningful prediction. Additionally, the method looks for features like important pixels in an image that is predictive of a class, and it finds a smaller subset of features that differentiate between the original instance and the predicted class.

3.10. Kernel Shapley

Kernel-SHAP deviates more efficiently, but not as precisely. Instead of doing randomised permutations of the features, we can simply use the model that has already been learned. In that, we find features to have equal "absent value" to equal "random value from data" [113]. When we realise that features don't have equal significance in the world" or "importance" with the new features, it has taken into account the Shapley values [113].

3.11. Integrated Gradients

Thesealso known as Path-Integrated Gradients or Axiomatic Attribution for Deep Networks. It gives an important feature-specific value to each input. Each insight can be explained with examples from personal experience. It is simple to implement and can be used on a wide range of datasets, like text datasets, images, and unstructured models like regression.It is an XAI technique that gives an important value to each feature of the input using the gradients of the model output [114].

3.12. Meta-Explanations

Finally, classification can be applied to individuals, allowing one to discover patterns across all classifiers. The newly developed meta-reasoning technique, spectral relevance analysis (SpRAy), uses heatmaps to determine their associations [115]. This approach allows analysis of the classifier's strategy on the entire dataset as well as the semi-automatic approach of fixing model/datasets when it shows bad results.

3.13. Software

Open-source software packages have dramatically increased the accessibility and credibility of both software research and deep learning in recent years. To make the method more accessible, the LRP toolbox [116] includes Python and MATLAB versions of the method as well as integration into the TensorFlow. The iNNvestigate toolbox [117] provides implements many of effective propagation-based explanation methods. One can often find these widely-used toolboxes below:

3.14. Interpret

Established by InterpretML for explaining the black-box models; this tool supports explainable boosting, decision trees, decision rule list, linear logistic regression, SHAP kernel explainer, SHAP tree explainer, LIME, sensitivity analysis, and partial dependence.

3.15. IML Package

It is maintained by Christoph Molnar [118, 119]. The package concealments feature importance, partial dependence plots, in addition to LIME, conditional plotting, accumulated local effects, tree surrogates, and SHAP.

3.16. DeepExplain

Marco Ancona maintains it [120]. It embodies different packages like gradient-based techniques such as saliency maps, gradient input, integrated gradients, DeepLIFT, LRP, etc., and perturbation-based methods such as occlusion, SHAP, etc.

3.17. DrWhy

It is given by ModelOriented and is a package with several model agnostic and model-specific XAI techniques, including feature importance, ceteris paribus, partial dependency plots, conditional dependency, etc.

4. Framework for Interpreting Explicability and Trust in Health Care

We currently have six important characteristics as empirical formulations for the explanation. This is in contrast to when people seek clarification as a reference to something else. The second reason is that definitions vary according to the focus of the question. People usually select one or two causes from a variety of possible causes as explanations. Using his or her personal and professional knowledge, the consumer decides on the causes he or she believes can help them. Explaining something to someone is an exchange; therefore, it's social. People want to know what the facts are and explanations to be truthful and complete. With people, it is generally preferred that explanations be easier and more generic. A comprehensive system of general trustworthiness and appropriate AI for health care purposes. The framework for interpreting explicability in health care consists of two components, as depicted in Figure 4: explanation characteristic and human-machine trust. Cognitive trust is impaired by the way machines, and affect-based trust is lost because of them. Although many previous research studies have established the necessity of human-to-to-human and machine-to-to-human trust, machine trust was derived from a study of computer trust. We have yet to determine whether there is a relationship between the two, but they have already been put in place.

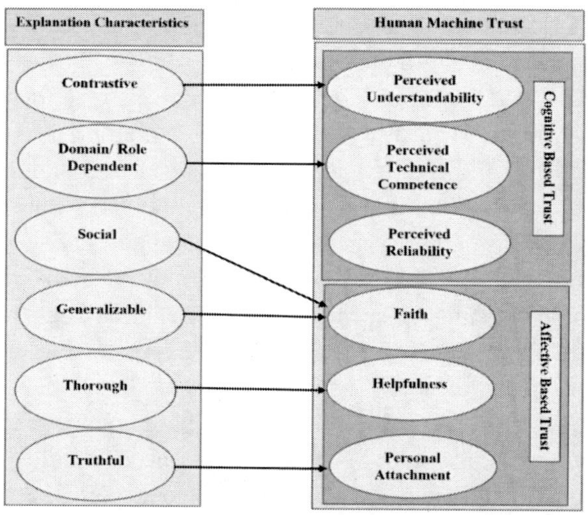

Figure 4. Trustworthy Explainable AI in Health care Framework.

5. Quality Evaluating of Explanations in Biomedical Domain

Does all learned models possess the same level of interpretability? Doshi-Vandelez and Kim [121] propose three interpretations of interpretability analysis (i) application-grounded (experiments with end-users): put your concept into practice and let the end user experiment with it. This type computes an explanation's quality according to its usefulness in achieving the end goal. (ii) human-grounded (experiments with lay humans): This approach treats the public as an integral part of the scientific process, in which experiments with the public are used, instead of trying to work with experts that isolate them from the general population. This one should be used when general notions of quality are being tested, and (iii) functionality-grounded evaluation (proxies based on a formal definition of interpretability): involves the regularisers that have already been grounded, like experiments or simulation. Despite the growing body of research, quantitative ML research results are few and difficult to measure; it is worth trying nonetheless (only 5 percent of the studied papers focus on this issue). As one observer has suggested, perhaps the subjectivity of explainability has something to do with it. However, because there are numerous interpretation methods already in existence, the requirement for comparing, validating, and quantifying them arises.

Perturbation analysis is commonly used to measure the quality of heatmaps [122]. According to the heatmap, the assumed effect of altering variables that are relevant to the solution (according to the heat) has a greater impact on its prediction than inputs that have a lesser effect. Explanation-based perturbations such as uniform noise should be used to enable comparisons between different methods but have been found to be inferior in other method quality criteria [122]. This technique has been used in several other studies to measure heatmaps like ""pointing gam" [123]. The goal of this game is to find the location of the category-relevant point in the heatmap. Proposals for evaluating tasks in the literature have been introduced, for example, to evaluate the design and creative efforts. Using the subject-verb agreement as an example [124]. In addition, the model predicts a verb number and determines the correct subject of the word based on the predictions. Other models of evaluation use intuition. On the other hand, a study [125] proposes to use data-driven theory to provide a relative explanation for sequential information. Thus, the authors of [127] have created word-level document representations. A document-level representation's performance (e.g., in a document classification task) is an indication of the quality of the category level explanations it embodies. According to this work, a new approach to reinforcement learning has been discovered. Instead of utilising arguments about whether or not functionalism has applications, a large number of scientifically and pragmatically-oriented statements [128] could be created that pertain to teaching and learning. A promising way to test theories is based on the fulfillment of an axiom [129].

5.1. How to Choose amongst Different Explainable AI Methods?

The search for best explainable artificial intelligence is a great challenge for domains where explainability is useful. This section is a resource for developers who need to learn how to design medical or caregiving AI systems. The type of explainability that may be important for different purposes can vary between different levels of complexity. Examine some of the difficulties a tradeoff that designers face while creating AI systems here. According to the criteria that can be applied to explainable AI methods, and in accordance with these findings, applied evaluations are less objective than the results that depend on human demographics. Qualitative and quantitative experimentation can be used in the same human experiments. A qualitative measurement takes into consideration things like relevance, usefulness, and trust in the interviews and questionnaires given. "Accuracy," "time needed to complete the task," "likelihood of error," and "ability to detect errors" are all quantitative measures of effectiveness. Applied evaluation provides the strongest evidence of success but can be inefficient because it is also repeated over and over time. Human studies are useful and necessary but also time-consuming and experimental.

5.1.1. Evaluating Model-Based Explanations

Fidelity of model-based explanations guarantees us that they are able to compute the result with an input model. Similarly, the task model of explainable modelling indicates that soundness is satisfied when the task is used as an explanation. Model-based explanations like those suggested by Lakkaraj et al. [130] can help us determine Fidelity. The definition of Fidelity is the amount of agreement between the task model and the post-hoc model. We contend that, in most cases, global descriptions aid comprehension as these methods provides one solution to the overall problem. Thus, the authors took into account the overlap of rules and feature space to define an unambiguous measurement in this instance. Our review could not find a clearness metric for model-based descriptions. To date, most model-explanation techniques tend to prefer using parsimony. There is a relationship between the model size and the level of model complexity [131]. Examples of measurable things are like number of features (e.g., non-zero weights, or number of rules) and tree depth, but they are both model-specific and model-dependent. Recently, Friedler et al. [132] suggested using operation counts (e.g., for calculating Boolean and arithmetic operations) to describe model complexity. They instead took a different approach and came up with an equation that utilises features and the magnitude of the main effect.

5.1.2. Evaluating Attribution-Based Explanations

When we go with the hypothesis of Fidelity, this only provides a partial explanation of the model, and therefore is not a full account. Various methods have been suggested in the literature, and we believe that soundness can be measured by using multiple methods. Ground truth is used to measure how well the method is performing, whereas scientific evaluation studies monitor the accuracy of the assertion through artificial measurement [134]. The performance-degrading technique involves using perturbation [135]. Some researchers adopt axiomatic approaches to try to see if certain properties of theories' turn-of-the-the-century conceptions of explanation hold. To answer the question of whether the answer (to the analysis) has something to do with the input, Kindermans and Hooker put forth a test that is sensitive to a meaningless transformation of the input data [136]. Sensitivity and implementation invariance were studied in [137] et al. Montavon et al. [138] describe this as the importance of continuity and selectivity. Ancona et al. [139] argue that an attribution method satisfies cardinality N when the total variation of cardinality is zero. This property is also called completeness or summation to the delta. Sadly, the two methods have their own set of serious issues. Although empirical methods describe what an attribution model should be capable of, they cannot distinguish task performance from results A different method, on the other hand, is difficult to define because of its semi-automated nature, like the axiomatic approach.

5.1.3. Evaluating Example-Based Explanations

Example-based evaluation methods are not found. Since the techniques differ according to objective (e.g., selecting prototypes, explaining influence, identifying vulnerabilities) and methods are limited, so are the evaluations. From these previous findings, we deduce that global explanations are both clear and necessary, whereas specific examples are parsimonious as long as they are understandable. Not a single method was found that would satisfy all of the remaining properties.

5.2. XAI Evaluating Measurements

The research community has suggested several evaluation schemes over the last few years. Current approaches that are in use:

5.2.1. System Causability Scale (SCS)

It is also important to consider how explainability methods are applied to human-facing AI, as evaluation of interfaces that use such systems becomes harder. The notion of a System Causability Scale (SCS) [140] was applied to the user-facing human-AI design to better explain the variables. A medical case in which the SCS was applied to the Framingham Risk Tool (FRT) was described as an opportunity to better understand how various characteristics of the human-AI interface impact outcomes.

5.2.2. Benchmarking Attribution Methods (BAM)

A Benchmarking Attribution Methods (BAM) for assessing the importance of various attributional features is suggested in work [141]. In this example, the BAM dataset is generated by duplicating feature groups called Common Features (CF), representing object categories from MSCOCO dataset [142], and pasting it into MiniPlaces dataset [43]. According to this theory, if the model contains the same pixel group of information at all locations, it is to be discounted as a significant feature. Because pasted features can' attempt to identify features that are doing a poor job, they do not apply successful ones. Model contrast score (MCS) served as the function to quantify the attribute degree of feature importance in terms of variance, input dependence rate (IDR) aimed to determine the variance of a single instance, and input independence rate (IIR) to determine how many regions have features attributions $g_r \in \square$ for the region r with and without CF is less than a set threshold.

5.2.3. Faithfulness and Monotonicity

Authors in [144] proposed a metric, known as Faithfulness, for rating the correlation between feature importance and the influence a feature has on performance. By removing the important features one at a little at a time to measure the relevance of the next one that is left. The authors in [145] introduced monadic functions, which focus on the performance of the model by progressively adding the more important individual features in sequence. Adding new and exciting features is expected to increase the performance of the model.

5.2.4. Human-Grounded Evaluation Benchmark

Moshseni et al. [146] empirically evaluated the local explanations by a XAI algorithm. The research employed humans to manually annotate a subset of the ImageNet dataset [147]. For purposes of comparison, a weighted representation of the explanations was generated, which showed an average human being. According to the explanations generated, a method was developed to evaluate the precision of XAI explanations in human terms. A major disadvantage of this method is that it may incorporate human error in the explanations. However, biases in a large sample of data may not hold true for the individuals who carry those labels.

5.3. Some Existing Real-Time Case Studies on XAI in Health Care

i): The work [148] designed an explainable AI early warning system (xAI-EWS) to monitor the health of patients. It incorporates a state-of-the-art, model for predicting sepsis from electronic health records (EHRs). The temporal convolution network (TC) and deep Taylor decomposition (DTD) prediction system is implemented here. The authors present results from three emergency medicine cases: sepsis, acute kidney injury (AKI), and acute lung injury (ALI). The xAI-EWS shows a high predictive performance while enabling the possibility to explain the predictions in terms of pinpointing decisive input data to empower clinicians to better understand the reasoning behind the predictions.

5.3.1. Predictive Performance

The learning capability of the xAI-EWS is displayed by evaluating it with results from the onset time to 24 h before onset. Area under the receiver operating characteristic curve (AUROC) with mean values and 95% confidence intervals (CIs) over the five cross-validations folds were 0.92 (0.9–0.95)–0.8 (0.78–83), 0.88 (0.86–0.9)–0.79 (0.78–0.8), and 0.90 (0.89–0.92)–0.84 (0.82–0.85) for sepsis, AKI, and ALI, respectively. Area under the precision-recall curve (AUPRC) with mean values and 95% CIs were 0.43 (0.36–0.51)–0.08 (0.07-0.09), 0.22 (0.19–0.24)–0.13 (0.12–0.14), and 0.23 (0.21–0.26)–0.23 (0.22–0.24) for sepsis, AKI, and ALI, respectively.

5.3.2. Explanations

With the xAI-EW models, we got two viewpoints on the model explanations: the individual viewpoint and a population view. A viewer tailored to the individual's needs provided explanation led the xAI to identify which clinical parameters were relevant at a given point in time. Under the current model, workflows normally proceed one of the two ways: high workload or an increase in workload. Targeted clinical intervention related to the development of a critical illness will be more effective if the clinician has an understanding of which clinical parameters are implicated in the current critical illness or its worsening. This is one of the main requirements for AI-based systems. The xAI-EWS system allows for explanations to be delivered in real-time and to be applied to all therapeutic parameters. Individual clinical parameters are calculated based on back-propagation of relevance. The best predictors of sepsis are a high respiration rate and low plasma albumin level. By inspection, it appears that the physiological relevance increases around the time of increased respiration frequency and pulse rate.

ii): The most important aspect of atrial fibrillation (AF) detection and management is early detection and intervention. Over the years, several diverse deep learning models (DLMs) have been developed but are not usable in clinical practice due to their inability to explain their findings. Authors [149], put up an innovative means of using DLM for AF unrevealing. The researchers used a saliency map to make their ECG more understandable. The inferences map only highlighted the relevant portions of the ECG and failed to explain the rationale for their existence. Also, for example, when we apply a deep learning algorithm to identify a QRS factor, we cannot understand what exactly is significant about the QRS complex. These DLM limitations were solved by incorporating state-of-the-art XAI methods like neural-backed ensemble tree (NBET). With an ECG-based DLM, the authors were able to develop an explainable AF detection method that was able to discriminate various AF rhythms [149].

5.3.3. Methods and Results

The Sejong ECG dataset comprising 128,399 ECGs was employed to validate the explainable DLM. DLM was externally validated using data from 21,837, 10,605, and 8528 ECGs from PTB-XL, Chapman, and PhysioNet non-restricted datasets, respectively. The predictors were in digital ECG format, and the endpoints were in base ECG format. For internal and external validation of the DLM, the AUC of the DLM was 0.997–0.999. The AUCs of the DLMs with the VAEs were between 0.990 and 0.999. An AUC for features like rhythmicity and the absence of P-wave anomalies were calculated to be 0.96–0.3, respectively. Our DLM correctly and reliably detected AF using a wide variety of ECGs, explaining our reasons for doing so. The results showed that a computer program explainable artificial intelligence could be adopted to enhance the DLM's clinical practice.

Conclusion

Advances in statistical learning are encouraging, and new discoveries in the AI field add significant capabilities to the medical field, but they are only used in a limited fashion because of the lack of understandable results. There's no doubt that artificial intelligence will play a significant role in health care. When you consider what humans are unable to do, AI has amazing potential. Despite the complexity of contemporary models, however: contemporary models are still considered to be "black box." The lack of detail makes it difficult for subject matter experts to understand why such a certain result has been obtained. As a result, the XAI community has developed a wide range of approaches to address such issues. This is a strong beginning, but we must push on to achieve better results (e.g., heatmaps). A human expert is usually needed to be brought in here because context is always important. The interactivity of human-machine interactions is required, specifically in the medical arena, in which numerous modalities come together to produce the result. XAI methods can be applied to systems derived from AI to explain the results. There are certain issues with the incorporation of XAI techniques. In order for XAI to be used in other health care systems, it needs to be constantly improved and expanded so that it can reach greater users and functions.

However, in contrast to white-box models, which are better able to catch nonlinearities and interactions between features, the black-box models perform poorly due to a lack of explainability. However, the less performing white-box models have observable/understandable features and relationships between variables and the output but do not always yield correct predictions (i.e., lower accuracy but higher explainability).

Being able to extract explanations of black-box model predictions is vital for the higher-risk endeavors in machine learning; this can be used to discriminate between black-box and color predictions in that realm. Localization offers new incidents to communicate to knowledgeable expert in the field of the domain. Human experts could benefit from this tertiary layer of knowledge. We need to further engage the developers, health care professionals, and lawmakers on this topic to address the challenges and limitations of opaque algorithms in the medical AI system.

References

Alber, M., Lapuschkin, S., Seegerer, P., H¨agele, M., Sch¨utt, K.T., Montavon, G., Samek, W., M¨uller, K.R., D¨ahne, S., Kindermans, P.J., iNNvestigate neural networks!. *Journal of Machine Learning Research* 20(93), 1–8 (2019).

Al-Shedivat, Maruan, Avinava Dubey, and Eric P. Xing" Contextual Explanation Networks" arXiv preprint arXiv:1705.10301 (2017).

Amina Adadi And Mohammed Berrada, "Peeking Inside the Black-Box: A Survey on Explainable Artificial Intelligence (XAI)," Volume 6, 2018, P.P.P., 52138- 52160.

Ancona, M., Ceolini, E., Oztireli, C., Gross, M., Gradient-based attribution methods. In: *Explainable AI: Interpreting, Explaining and Visualising Deep Learning. Lecture Notes in Computer Science* 11700, Springer (2019).

Ancona, M., E. Ceolini, C. Oztireli, ¨ M. Gross, Towards better understanding of gradient-based attribution methods for deep neural networks [Preprint]. March 7, 2018. https://arxiv.org/abs/1711.06104.

Ancona, M., E. Ceolini, C. Oztireli, and M. Gross, "Towards better ¨ understanding of gradient-based attribution methods for deep neural networks," 6th International Conference on Learning Representations, ICLR 2018 - Conference Track Proceedings, 2018.

Aniek F. Markus, Jan A. Kors, and Peter R. Rijnbeek, "The role of explainability in creating trustworthy artificial intelligence for health care: A comprehensive survey of the terminology, design choices, and evaluation strategies," *Journal of Biomedical Informatics,* Volume 113, January 2021, 103655, pp: 1-11.

Aniek F. Markus, Jan A. Kors, and Peter R. Rijnbeek, "The role of explainability in creating trustworthy artificial intelligence for health care: A comprehensive survey of the terminology, design choices, and evaluation strategies," *Journal of Biomedical Informatics,* Volume 113, 2021, 103655, pp: 1-11.

Arjona-Medina, J. A., Gillhofer, M., Widrich, M., Unterthiner, T., Hochreiter, S., RUDDER: Return Decomposition for Delayed Rewards. arXiv preprint arXiv:1806. 07857 (2018).

Arras, L., A. Osman, K. R. Müller, W. Samek, Evaluating recurrent neural network explanations [Preprint]. June 4, 2019. https://arxiv.org/abs/1904.11829.

Arras, L., Arjona-Medina, J., Gillhofer, M., Widrich, M., Montavon, G., M¨uller, K. R., Hochreiter, S., Samek, W., Explaining and interpreting LSTMs with LRP. In: *Explainable AI: Interpreting, Explaining and Visualising Deep Learning. Lecture Notes in Computer Science* 11700, pp. 211238. Springer (2019).

Arras, L., Horn, F., Montavon, G., M¨uller, K.R., Samek, W., "What is relevant in a text document?": An interpretable machine learning approach. *PLoS ONE* 12(8), e0181142 (2017).

Arras, L., Osman, A., Muller, K.R., Samek, W., Evaluating recurrent neural network explanations. In: *ACL'19 Workshop on BlackboxNLP: Analysing and Interpreting Neural Networks for NLP,* pp. 113-126 (2019).

Arun Das, and Paul Rad, "Opportunities and Challenges in Explainable Artificial Intelligence (XAI): A Survey," arXiv:2006.11371v2 [cs.CV] 23 Jun 2020.

Bach, S., A. Binder, G. Montavon, F. Klauschen, K. R. Müller, and W. Samek. On pixel-wise explanations for non-linear classifier decisions by layer-wise relevance propagation. *PLoS ONE,* 10(7):e0130140, 2015.

Baehrens, D., T. Schroeter, S. Harmeling, M. Kawanabe, K. Hansen, and K.-R. Müller, "How to explain individual classi_cation decisions," *J. Mach. Learn. Res.*, vol. 11, no. 6, pp. 1803_1831, 2010.

Bahdanau, D., Cho, K., Bengio, Y., Neural machine translation by jointly learning to align and translate. In: *International Conference on Learning Representations (ICLR).* (2015).

Barocas, S., S. Friedler, M. Hardt, J. Kroll, S. Venka-Tasubramanian, and H. Wallach. The FAT-ML Workshop Series on Fairness, Accountability, and Transparency in Machine Learning. Accessed: Jun. 6, 2018. [Online]. Available: http://www.fatml.org/.

Bastani, O., C. Kim, and H. Bastani. (2017). "Interpretability via model extraction." [Online]. Available: https://arxiv.org/abs/1706.09773.

Benjamin Letham, Cynthia Rudin, Tyler H. McCormick, and David Madigan. Interpretable classifiers using rules and bayesian analysis: Building a better stroke prediction model. *The Annals of Applied Statistics,* 9(3):13501371, Sep 2015.

Caruana, R., Y. Lou, J. Gehrke, P. Koch, M. Sturm, and N. Elhadad, "Intelligible models for health care: Predicting pneumonia risk and hospital 30-day readmission" in *Proc. 21th ACM SIGKDD Int. Conf. Knowl. Discovery Data Mining,* 2015, pp. 1721–1730.

Caruana, R., Y. Lou, J. Gehrke, P. Koch, M. Sturm, and N. Elhadad, "Intelligible models for health care: Predicting pneumonia risk and hospital 30-day readmission," in *Proc. 21th ACM SIGKDD Int. Conf. Knowl. Discovery Data Mining*, 2015, pp. 1721_1730.

Caruana, Rich, Yin Lou, Johannes Gehrke, Paul Koch, Marc Sturm, and Noemie Elhadad. "Intelligible models for health care: Predicting pneumonia risk and hospital 30-day readmission." In *Proceedings of the 21th ACM SIGKDD International Conference on Knowledge Discovery and Data Mining,* pp. 1721-1730. ACM, 2015.

Che, Z., S. Purushotham, R. Khemani, and Y. Liu. (2015). "Distilling knowledge from deep networks with applications to health care domain." [Online]. Available: https://arxiv.org/abs/1512.03542.

Ciresan, D., Meier, U., Masci, J., Schmidhuber, J., A committee of neural networks for traffic sign classification. In: *International Joint Conference on Neural Networks (IJCNN).* pp. 1918–1921 (2011).

Cook, R. D., Detection of influential observation in linear regression, Technometrics 19 (1977) 15–18, https://doi.org/10.1080/00401706.1977.10489493.

Deng, J., W. Dong, R. Socher, L. Li, Kai Li, and Li Fei-Fei, "Imagenet: A large-scale hierarchical image database," in *2009 IEEE Conference on Computer Vision and Pattern Recognition,* 2009, pp. 248–255.

Devam Dave, Het Naik, Smiti Singhal, and Pankesh Patel, "Explainable AI meets Health care: A Study on Heart Disease Dataset," arXiv:2011.03195v1 [cs.LG] 6 Nov 2020, p: 1-13.

Dibben, M. R., Lean, M., Achieving compliance in chronic illness management: illustrations of trust relationships between physicians and nutrition clinic patients. *Health, Risk & Society* 5(3), 241-258 (2003).

Doilovi£, F. K., M. Br£i¢, and N. Hlupi¢, "Explainable arti_cial intelligence: A survey," in *Proc. 41st Int. Conv. Inf. Commun. Technol., Electron. Microelectron.* (MIPRO), May 2018, pp. 0210_0215.

Doshi-Velez 2014 Doshi-Velez, Finale, and Been Kim. "Towards a rigorous science of interpretable machine learning." arXiv preprint arXiv:1702.08608 (2017).

Doshi-Velez, F., and B. Kim, "Towards A Rigorous Science of Interpretable Machine Learning" no. Ml, pp. 1–13, 2017.

Doshi-Velez, F., and B. Kim. (2018). "Towards a rigorous science of interpretable machine learning." [Online]. Available: https://arxiv.org/abs/1702.08608.

Doshi-Velez, F., Kim, B., Towards a rigorous science of interpretable machine learning. arXiv preprint arXiv:1702.08608 (2017).

Doshi-Velez, F., Kim, B., Towards a rigorous science of interpretable machine learning. arXiv preprint arXiv:1702.08608 (2017).

Erdem Varol, Aristeidis Sotiras, Ke Zeng, and Christos Davatzikos. Generative discriminative models for multivariate inference and statistical mapping in medical imaging. In Alejandro F. Frangi, Julia A. Schnabel, Christos Davatzikos, Carlos Alberola-Lopez, and Gabor' Fichtinger, editors, Medical Image Computing and Computer Assisted Intervention – MICCAI 2018, pages 540–548, Cham, 2018. Springer International Publishing.

Erico Tjoa, and Cuntai Guan, F, "A Survey on Explainable Artificial Intelligence (XAI): towards Medical XAI," *Journal of Latex Class Files,* VOL. 14, NO. 8, AUGUST 2015, pp: 1-11.

Everingham, M., Van Gool, L., Williams, C.K., Winn, J., Zisserman, A., The Pascal visual object classes (VOC) challenge. *International Journal of Computer Vision* 88(2), 303–338 (2010).

Faust, Kevin, Bala, Sudarshan, Van Ommeren, Randy, Portante, Alessia, Al Qawahmed, Raniah, Djuric, Ugljesa & Diamandis, Phedias 2019. Intelligent feature engineering and ontological mapping of brain tumour histomorphologies by deep learning. *Nature Machine Intelligence,* 1, (7), 316–321, doi:10.1038/s42256-019-0068-6.

FICO. (2018). Explainable Machine Learning Challenge. Accessed: Jun. 6, 2018. [Online]. Available: https://community.fico.com/s/explainable-machine-learning-challenge.

Fong, R. C., Vedaldi, A., Interpretable explanations of black boxes by meaningful perturbation. In: *IEEE International Conference on Computer Vision (CVPR).* pp. 3429–3437 (2017).

Fong, R., Vedaldi, A., Explanations for attributing deep neural network predictions. In: *Explainable AI: Interpreting, Explaining and Visualising Deep Learning. Lecture Notes in Computer Science* 11700, pp. 149167. Springer (2019).

Friedler, S. A., C. D. Roy, C. Scheidegger, D. Slack, *Assessing the local interpretability of machine learning models* [Preprint]. August 2, 2019. https://arxiv.org/abs/1902.03501.

Gold, C., et al. Trust in Automation Before and After the Experience of Take-over Scenarios in a Highly Automated Vehicle." In: *Procedia Manufacturing* Volume 3, 2015, Pages 3025-3032 (2015). doi: https://doi.org/10.1016/j.promfg.2015.07.847.

Guidotti, R., A. Monreale, S. Ruggieri, F. Turini, F. Giannotti, D. Pedreschi, A survey of methods for explaining black box models, *ACM Computing Surveys* (CSUR) 51 (2018) 93, https://doi.org/10.1145/3236009.

Gunning, D., Explainable articial intelligence (xai) (2017).

Gunning, D., Explainable artificial intelligence (XAI), Defense Advanced Research Projects Agency (DARPA). Accessed: Jun. 6, 2018. [Online]. Available: http://www.darpa.mil/program/explainable-artificialintelligence.

Han, S., Pool, J., Tran, J., Dally, W., Learning both weights and connections for efficient neural network. In: *Advances in Neural Information Processing Systems* (NIPS). pp. 1135–1143 (2015).

Harsha Nori et al. InterpretML: A Uni_ed Framework for Machine Learning Interpretability." In: arXiv preprint arXiv:1909.09223 (2019).

Henelius, A., K. Puolamäki, and A. Ukkonen. (2017). "Interpreting classifiers through attribute interactions in datasets" [Online]. Available: https://arxiv.org/abs/1707.07576.

Holzinger, A., A. Carrington, and H. M¨uller, "Measuring the Quality of Explanations: The System Causability Scale (SCS)," K.K.I. - Kunstliche Intelligenz, pp. 193–198, 2020.

Holzinger, Andreas, Langs, Georg, Denk, Helmut, Zatloukal, Kurt & Müller, Heimo 2019. Causability and Explainability of Artifcial Intelligence in Medicine. Wiley Interdisciplinary Reviews: Data Mining and Knowledge Discovery, 9, (4), 1–13, doi:10.1002/widm.1312.

Hyebin Lee, Seong Tae Kim, and Yong Man Ro. Generation of multimodal justification using visual word constraint model for explainable computer-aided diagnosis. In Kenji Suzuki, Mauricio Reyes, Tanveer Syeda-Mahmood, Ben Glocker, Roland Wiest, Yaniv Gur, Hayit Greenspan, and Anant Madabhushi, editors, Interpretability of Machine Intelligence in Medical Image Computing and Multimodal Learning for Clinical Decision Support, pages 21–29, Cham, 2019. Springer International Publishing.

Jamie A. Duell, "A Comparative Approach to Explainable Arti_cial Intelligence (XAI) Methods in Application to High-Dimensional Electronic Health Records: Examining the Usability of XAI," arXiv:2103.04951v1 [cs. L. L.G.] 8 Mar 2021.pp: 1-18.

Karpathy, A., Toderici, G., Shetty, S., Leung, T., Sukthankar, R., Fei-Fei, L., Largescale video classification with convolutional neural networks. In: *IEEE conference on Computer Vision and Pattern Recognition (CVPR).* pp. 1725–1732 (2014).

Khedkar, S., V. Subramanian, G. Shinde, and P. Gandhi, "Explainable AI in Health care," *SSRN Electronic Journal,* 2019.

Kim, B., R. Khanna, O. O. Koyejo, Examples are not enough, learn to criticise! Criticism for interpretability, *Adv. Neural Inform. Process. Syst.* 29 (2016) 2280–2288.

Knight, W., (2017). The US military wants its autonomous machines to explain themselves, *MIT Technology Review.* Accessed: Jun. 6, 2018. [Online]. Available: https://www.technologyreview.com/s/603795/theus-military-wants-its-autonomous-machines-to-explain-themselves.

Lakkaraju, H., E. Kamar, R. Caruana, J. Leskovec, *Interpretable & explorable approximations of black box models* [Preprint]. July 4, 2017. https://arxiv.org/pdf/1707.01154.pdf.

Lakkaraju, H., S. H. Bach, and J. Leskovec,"Interpretable decision sets: A joint framework for description and prediction" *Proceedings of the ACM SIGKDD International Conference on Knowledge Discovery and Data Mining,* vol. 13-17-August-2016, pp. 1675–1684, 2016.

Lakkaraju, Himabindu, Kamar, Ece, Caruana, Rich & Leskovec, Jure 2017. Interpretable and Explorable Approximations of Black Box Models. arXiv:1707.01154.

Lapuschkin, S., A. Binder, G. Montavon, K. R. Müller, and W. Samek. Analysing classifiers: Fisher vectors and deep neural networks. In *Proceedings of the IEEE Conference on Computer Vision and Pattern Recognition (CVPR),* pages 2912–2920, 2016.

Lapuschkin, S., Binder, A., Montavon, G., M¨uller, K.R., Samek, W., Analysing classifiers: Fisher vectors and deep neural networks. In: *IEEE Conference on Computer Vision and Pattern Recognition (CVPR).* pp. 2912–2920 (2016).

Lapuschkin, S., Binder, A., Montavon, G., M¨uller, K.R., Samek, W., Analysing classifiers: Fisher vectors and deep neural networks. In: *IEEE Conference on Computer Vision and Pattern Recognition (CVPR).* pp. 2912–2920 (2016).

Lapuschkin, S., Opening the Machine Learning Black Box with Layer-wise Relevance Propagation. Ph.D. thesis, Technische Universit¨at Berlin (2019).

Lapuschkin, S., W¨aldchen, S., Binder, A., Montavon, G., Samek, W., Muller, K. R., Unmasking clever hans predictors and assessing what machines really learn. *Nature Communications* 10, 1096 (2019).

Lapuschkin, S., Waldchen, S., Binder, A., Montavon, G., Samek, W., M¨uller, K. R., Unmasking clever hans predictors and assessing what machines really learn. *Nature Communications* 10, 1096 (2019).

LeCun, Y. A., Bottou, L., Orr, G. B., M¨uller, K. R., Efficient backprop. In: *Neural networks: Tricks of the trade,* pp. 9–48. Springer (2012).

Lei, J., M. G'Sell, A. Rinaldo, R. J. Tibshirani, and L. Wasserman, "Distribution-free predictive inference for regression," *J. Amer. Stat. Assoc.*, to be published. [Online]. Available: http://www.stat.cmu.edu/~ryantibs/papers/conformal.pdf.

Letham, B., C. Rudin, T. H. McCormick, and D. Madigan, "Interpretable classiers using rules and Bayesian analysis: Building a better stroke prediction model," *Ann. Appl. Statist.*, vol. 9, no. 3, pp. 1350_1371, 2015.

Lightbourne, J., "Damned lies & criminal sentencing using evidencebased tools" 15 Duke Law & Technol. *Rev., Tech. Rep.*, 2017, pp. 327–343. Accessed: Jun. 6, 2018. https://scholarship.law.duke.edu/ dltr/vol15/iss1/16.

Lin, T. Y., M. Maire, S. Belongie, J. Hays, P. Perona, D. Ramanan, P. Doll'ar, and C. L. Zitnick, "Microsoft coco: Common objects in context," in European conference on computer vision. Springer, 2014, pp. 740–755.

Lindholm, E., Nickolls, J., Oberman, S., Montrym, J., Nvidia tesla: A unified graphics and computing architecture. *IEEE Micro* 28(2), 39–55 (2008).

Looveren, A. V., Klaise, J., Interpretable counterfactual explanations guided by prototypes (2020).

Loyola-Gonzalez, O. Black-Box vs. White-Box: Understanding Their Advantages and Weaknesses From a Practical Point of View." In: (2019). doi: 10.1109/ACCESS.2019.2949286.

Lundberg, S. M., and S. I. Lee, "A unified approach to interpreting model predictions," in *Advances in neural information processing systems,* pp. 4765–4774, 2017.

Lundberg, S. M., Lee, S. I., A unified approach to interpreting model predictions. In: *Advances in neural information processing systems.* pp. 4765–4774 (2017).

Lundberg, S. M., Lee, S. I., A unified approach to interpreting model predictions. In: *Advances in neural information processing systems.* pp. 4765–4774 (2017).

Lundberg, S., H. Chen and S. Lee. Explaining Models by Propagating Shapley Values." In: arXiv:1911.11888 (2019).

Luss, R., P. Y. Chen, A. Dhurandhar, P. Sattigeri, K. Shanmugam, and C.-C. Tu, "Generating contrastive explanations with monotonic attribute functions," arXiv preprint arXiv:1905.12698, 2019.

Madry, A., Makelov, A., Schmidt, L., Tsipras, D., Vladu, A., Towards deep learning models resistant to adversarial attacks. In: *International Conference on Learning Representations (ICLR).* (2018).

McFarland, M., (2018). Uber Shuts Down Self-Driving Operations in Arizona, CNN. Accessed Jun. 6, 2018. [Online]. Available: http://money.cnn.com/2018/05/23/technology/uber-arizona-selfdriving/index.html.

Melis, D. A., and T. Jaakkola, "Towards robust interpretability with self-explaining neural networks," in *Advances in Neural Information Processing Systems,* 2018, pp. 7775–7784.

Meyer Lauritsen, Simon, Mads Kristensen, Mathias Vassard Olsen, Morten Skaarup Larsen, Katrine Meyer Lauritsen, Marianne Johansson Jorgensen, Jeppe Lange and Bo Thiesson, "Explainable artificial intelligence model to predict acute critical illness from electronic health records," *Nature Communications,* (2020) 11:3852, 1-11.

Mohseni, S., and E. D. Ragan, "A human-grounded evaluation benchmark for local explanations of machine learning," arXiv preprint arXiv:1801.05075, 2018.

Molnar, C., G. Casalicchio, and B. Bischl, "iml: An r package for interpretable machine learning," *Journal of Open Source Software,* vol. 3, no. 26, p. 786, 2018.

Molnar, C., G. Casalicchio, B. Bischl, Quantifying interpretability of arbitrary machine learning models through functional decomposition [Preprint]. September 23, 2019. https://arxiv.org/pdf/1904.03867.pdf.

Molnar, C., Interpretable Machine Learning. Lulu. com, 2020.

Montavon, G., Binder, A., Lapuschkin, S., Samek, W., Muller, K.R., Layer-wise relevance propagation: An overview. In: *Explainable AI: Interpreting, Explaining and Visualising Deep Learning. Lecture Notes in Computer Science* 11700, pp. 193-209. Springer (2019).

Montavon, G., S. Bach, A. Binder, W. Samek, and K. R. Müller. Explaining non-linear classification decisions with deep taylor decomposition. *Pattern Recognition,* 65:211–222, 2017.

Montavon, G., S. Lapuschkin, A. Binder, W. Samek, and K.-R. Müller, "Explaining non-linear classi_cation decisions with deep taylor decomposition," *Pattern Recognit.*, vol. 65, pp. 211_222, May 2017.

Montavon, G., S. Lapuschkin, A. Binder, W. Samek, K.-R. Müller, Explaining non-linear classification decisions with deep taylor decomposition, Pattern Recognit. 65 (2017) 211–222, https://doi.org/10.1016/j.patcog.2016.11.008.

Montavon, G., W. Samek, K.-R. Müller, Methods for interpreting and understanding deep neural networks, *Digit. Signal Process.* 73 (2018) 1–15, https://doi.org/10.1016/j.dsp.2017.10.011.

Moravcık, M., Schmid, M., Burch, N., Lisy, V., Morrill, D., Bard, N., et al. Deepstack: Expert-level artificial intelligence in heads-up no-limit poker. *Science* 356(6337), 508–513 (2017).

Mordvintsev, A., Olah, C., Tyka, M., Inceptionism: Going deeper into neural networks (2015).

Nguyen, A., Dosovitskiy, A., Yosinski, J., Brox, T., Clune, J., Synthesising the preferred inputs for neurons in neural networks via deep generator networks. In: *Advances in Neural Information Processing Systems (NIPS).* pp. 3387–3395 (2016).

Pawar, U., D. O. Shea, S. Rea, and R. O. Reilly, Incorporating Explainable Artificial Intelligence (XAI) to aid the Understanding of Machine Learning in the Health care Domain, CEUR-WS.org/vol. 2771/AISC2020_paper_62.pdf, pp: 1-12.

Pieter Van Molle, Miguel De Strooper, Tim Verbelen, Bert Vankeirsbilck, Pieter Simoens, and Bart Dhoedt. Visualising convolutional neural networks to improve decision support for skin lesion classification. In Danail Stoyanov, Zeike Taylor, Seyed Mostafa Kia, Ipek Oguz, Mauricio Reyes, Anne Martel, Lena Maier-Hein, Andre F. Marquand, Edouard Duchesnay, Tommy Lofstedt, Bennett Landman, ¨ M. Jorge Cardoso, Carlos A. Silva, Sergio Pereira, and Raphael Meier, editors, Understanding and Interpreting Machine Learning in Medical Image Computing Applications, pages 115–123, Cham, 2018. Springer International Publishing.

Poerner, N., Roth, B., Schutze, H., Evaluating neural network explanation methods using hybrid documents and morphosyntactic agreement. In: *56th Annual Meeting of the Association for Computational Linguistics (ACL).* pp. 340–350 (2018).

Rahim, Sarni Suhaila, Palade, Vasile, Almakky, Ibrahim & Holzinger, Andreas 2019. Detection of Diabetic Retinopathy and Maculopathy in Eye Fundus Images Using Deep Learning and Image Augmentation. International Cross-Domain Conference for Machine Learning and Knowledge Extraction. Springer, pp. 114–127, doi:10.1007/978-3-030-29726-8_8.

Redmon, J., Divvala, S., Girshick, R., Farhadi, A., You only look once: Unified, real-time object detection. In: *IEEE Conference on Computer Vision and Pattern Recognition (CVPR).* pp. 779–788 (2016).

Retno Larasati and Anna DeLiddo, "Building a Trustworthy Explainable AI in Health care," 1-8.

Ribeiro, M. T., and C. Guestrin, "Anchors: High-Precision Model-Agnostic Explanations."

Ribeiro, M. T., and C. Guestrin, "Why Should I Trust You ?" Explaining the Predictions of Any Classifier," pp. 1135– 1144, 2016.

Ribeiro, M. T., S. Singh, and C. Guestrin, "Anchors: High-precision model-agnostic explanations," in *Proc. AAAI Conf. Artif. Intell.*, 2018, pp. 1_9.

Ribeiro, M. T., S. Singh, and C. Guestrin, "Why should i trust you?': Explaining the predictions of any classier," in *Proc. 22nd ACM SIGKDD Int. Conf. Knowl. Discovery Data Mining*, 2016, pp. 1135_1144.

Ribeiro, M. T., Singh, S., Guestrin, C., Anchors: High-precision model-agnostic explanations. In: *AAAI Conference on Artificial Intelligence (AAAI)* (2018).

Ribeiro, M. T., Singh, S., Guestrin, C., Why should i trust you?: Explaining the predictions of any classifier. In: ACM SIGKDD International Conference on Knowledge Discovery and Data Mining. pp. 1135–1144 (2016).

Ribeiro, M. T., Singh, S., Guestrin, C., Why should i trust you?: Explaining the predictions of any classifier. In: *ACM SIGKDD International Conference on Knowledge Discovery and Data Mining.* pp. 1135–1144 (2016).

Rich Caruana, Yin Lou, Johannes Gehrke, Paul Koch, Marc Sturm, and Noemie Elhadad. Intelligible models for health care: Predicting pneumonia risk and hospital 30-day readmission. In Proceedings of the 21th ACM SIGKDD International Conference on Knowledge Discovery and Data Mining, KDD 15, page 17211730, New York, NY, USA, 2015. Association for Computing Machinery.

Robnik-Sikonja, M., and I. Kononenko, "Explaining classi_cations for individual instances," *IEEE Trans. Knowl. Data Eng.*, vol. 20, no. 5, pp. 589_600, May 2008.

Rudin, Cynthia 2019. Stop explaining black box machine learning models for high stakes decisions and use interpretable models instead. *Nature Machine Intelligence,* 1, (5), 206–215, doi:10.1038/s42256-019-0048-x.

S. Lapuschkin, A. Binder, G. Montavon, K. R. Müller, and W. Samek. The layer-wise relevance propagation toolbox for artificial neural networks. *Journal of Machine Learning Research,* 17(114):1–5, 2016.

Samek, W., Binder, A., Montavon, G., Lapuschkin, S., Muller, K.R., Evaluating the visualisation of what a deep neural network has learned. *IEEE Transactions on Neural Networks and Learning Systems* 28(11), 2660–2673 (2017).

Samek, W., Explainable AI: Interpreting, explaining and visualising deep learning: Springer Nature, 2019.

Shaikh, T. A. and Ali, R. (2020), "Computer-aided Big Health care Data (BHD) Analytics," Tanwar, P., Jain, V., Liu, C. M. and Goyal, V. (Ed.) Big Data Analytics and Intelligence: A Perspective for Health Care, Emerald Publishing Limited, Bingley, pp. 115-138. https://doi.org/10.1108/978-1-83909-099-820201010.

Shaikh, T. A., and R. Ali, "Applying machine learning algorithms for early diagnosis and prediction of breast cancer risk," in *Proceedings of 2nd International Conference on Communication, Computing and Networking* (ICCCN), Chandigarh India, Springer, Singapore, 2019, Pp:589-598.

Shaikh, T. A., R. Ali, & M. M. S. Beg, Transfer learning privileged information fuels CAD diagnosis of breast cancer. *Machine Vision and Applications,* 31, 9 (2020). Pp: 1-23.

Silver, D., Huang, A., Maddison, C. J., Guez, A., Sifre, L., Van Den Driessche, G., et al., Mastering the game of Go with deep neural networks and tree search. *Nature* 529(7587), 484–489 (2016).

Simonyan, K., A. Vedaldi, and A. Zisserman. Deep inside convolutional networks: Visualising image classification models and saliency maps. arXiv preprint arXiv:1312.6034, 2013.

Simonyan, K., Vedaldi, A., Zisserman, A., Deep inside convolutional networks: Visualising image classification models and saliency maps. In: *ICLR Workshop.* (2014).

Smilkov, D., Thorat, N., Kim, B., Vi'egas, F., Wattenberg, M., Smoothgrad: removing noise by adding noise. arXiv preprint arXiv:1706.03825 (2017).

Springenberg, J. T., Dosovitskiy, A., Brox, T., Riedmiller, M., Striving for simplicity: The all convolutional net. In: *ICLR Workshop.* (2015).

Sundararajan, M., A. Taly, Q. Yan, Axiomatic attribution for deep networks, in: Proceedings of the 34th International Conference on Machine Learning, 2017, pp. 3319–3328.

Sundararajan, M., Taly, A., Yan, Q., Axiomatic attribution for deep networks. In: *International Conference on Machine Learning (ICML).* pp. 3319–3328 (2017).

Sundararajan, M., Taly, A., Yan, Q., Axiomatic attribution for deep networks. arXiv preprint arXiv:1703.01365 (2017).

Sundararajan, M., Taly, A., Yan, Q., Axiomatic attribution for deep networks. In: *International Conference on Machine Learning (ICML).* pp. 3319–3328 (2017).

Tan, S., R. Caruana, G. Hooker, and Y. Lou. (2018). "Detecting bias in black-box models using transparent model distillation" [Online]. Available: https://arxiv.org/abs/1710.06169.

Thiagarajan, J. J., B. Kailkhura, P. Sattigeri, and K. N. Ramamurthy. (2016). "TreeView: Peeking into deep neural networks via feature-space partitioning." [Online]. Available: https://arxiv.org/abs/1611.07429.

Thomas, A. W., H. R. Heekeren, K. R. Muller, and W. Samek. Ana- ¨ lyzing Neuroimaging Data Through Recurrent Deep Learning Models. *Front Neurosci,* 13:1321, 2019.

Tonekaboni, S., et al. What Clinicians Want: Contextualizing Explainable Machin e Learning for Clinical End Use." In: arXiv preprint 1905.05134 (2019).

van Lent, M., W. Fisher, and M. Mancuso, "An explainable artificial intelligence system for small-unit tactical behavior" in *Proc. 16th Conf. Innov. Appl. Artif. Intell.,* 2004, pp. 900–907.

Vilamala, A., K. H. Madsen, and L. K. Hansen. Deep convolutional neural networks for interpretable analysis of eeg sleep stage scoring. In *2017 IEEE 27th International Workshop on Machine Learning for Signal Processing (MLSP),* pages 1–6, 2017.

Vishal Sharma, Piyush, Samarth Chhatwal, and Bipin Singh, "An Explainable Artificial Intelligence based Prospective Framework for COVID-19 Risk Prediction," Preprint March 5, 2021, https://doi.org/10.1101/2021.03.02.21252269.

Wachter, S., B. Mittelstadt, and C. Russell. (2017). "Counterfactual explanations without opening the black box: Automated decisions and the GDPR." [Online]. Available: https://arxiv.org/abs/1711.00399.

Wachter, S., Mittelstadt, B., Russell, C., Counterfactual explanations without opening the black box: Automated decisions and the gdpr (2018).

Wang, D., Q. Yang, A. Abdul, and B. Y. Lim, "Designing Theory-Driven User-Centric Explainable A. I. A. I.," *Proceedings of the 2019 CHI Conference on Human Factors in Computing Systems - CHI '19,* pp. 1–15, 2019.

Wu, D., Wang, L., Zhang, P., Solving statistical mechanics using variational autoregressive networks. *Physical Review Letters* 122(8), 080602 (2019).

Xu, K., D. H. Park, D. H. Yi, and C. Sutton. (2018). "Interpreting deep classi_er by visual distillation of dark knowledge." [Online]. Available: https://arxiv.org/abs/1803.04042.

Yang, C., A. Rangarajan, and S. Ranka. (2018). "*Global model interpretation via recursive partitioning.*" [Online]. Available: https://arxiv. org/abs/1802.04253.

Yang, M. and B. Kim, "Benchmarking Attribution Methods with Relative Feature Importance," CoRR, vol. abs/1907.09701, 2019.

Zeiler, M. D., Fergus, R., Visualising and understanding convolutional networks. In: *European Conference Computer Vision (ECCV).* pp. 818–833 (2014).

Zeiler, M. D., Fergus, R., Visualising and understanding convolutional networks. In: *European Conference Computer Vision (ECCV).* pp. 818–833 (2014).

Zhang, J., Lin, Z.L., Brandt, J., Shen, X., Sclaroff, S., Top-down neural attention by excitation backprop. In: *European Conference on Computer Vision (ECCV).* pp. 543–559 (2016).

Zhou, B., A. Lapedriza, A. Khosla, A. Oliva, and A. Torralba, "Places: A 10 Million Image Database for Scene Recognition," *IEEE Trans. Pattern Anal. Mach. Intell.,* vol. 40, no. 6, pp. 1452–1464, Jun 2018.

Zintgraf, L. M., Cohen, T. S., Adel, T., Welling, M., Visualising deep neural network decisions: Prediction difference analysis. In: *International Conference on Learning Representations (ICLR).* (2017).

Ziqi Tang, Kangway V. Chuang, Charles DeCarli, Lee-Way Jin, Laurel Beckett, Michael J. Keiser, and Brittany N. Dugger. Interpretable classification of alzheimer's disease pathologies with a convolutional neural network pipeline. *Nature Communications,* 10(1):2173, 2019.

Chapter 10

SleepEEG Study: Automated Sleep Stage System with Machine Learning Techniques

Santosh Kumar Satapathy[1,*], Debabrata Swain[2] and Rupalin Nanda[3]

[1]Department of Information and Communication Technology, Pandit Deendayal Energy University, Gujarat, India

[2]Department of Computer Science and Engineering, Pandit Deendayal Energy University, Gujarat, India

[3]Department of Department of Electronics and Communication Engineering, Anna University, Chennai, Tamil Nadu, India

Abstract

Electroencephalogram (EEG) is most acceptable in sleep disorder analysis. It is an essential primary signal through which we monitor the significant activities in the brain. It has been used to diagnose any sleep-related diseases. The manual sleep scoring approach is entirely not consistent with sleep scores from multiple sleep experts, and it has also taken more time for clinicians to complete the task. The main objective of this study is automatic sleep stage classification on dual channels of EEG signals in gender-specific subjects. In this study, we have considered four basic steps: i) pre-processing, ii) feature extraction, iii) feature selection, and iv) classification. This proposed, we have also considered some existing approaches, procedures, and methods to detect the abnormality in sleep states. Here we have combined the NREM and REM stages into one stage, called the sleep stage. Here we have proposed a two-stage classification. We have selected one public dataset of sleep study named ISRUC-Sleep dataset collected from the Hospital of Coimbra University (CHUC) in the sleep department in Portugal for this research work. In this study, we have considered two channels of EEG

[*]Corresponding Author's Email: Santosh.Satapathy@sot.pdpu.ac.in.

signals with different sex subjects. Feature selection and classifiers assess which channel recordings and which classification algorithm is more suitable for accurately discriminating the different sleep stages specific to subject and gender. In our proposed research work, the SVM classification techniques turned out to be most helpful in classifying the sleep stages of subject-16 through the C4-A1 channel with an accuracy of 97.20% and kappa coefficient of 1.88, similarly for the O2-A1 channel with an accuracy of 98.53% and kappa coefficient of 1.92, which indicates a substantial agreement with the gold standard. We have presented a novel comparison of channel effectiveness in the count to sleep scoring of sleep stages. We also compared classification algorithm performance in this study, and the results make it more suitable for scientific and clinical sleep disorder assessment.

1. Introduction

In this research paper, we have proposed the importance of sleep stage classification systems during the investigation of sleep-related disorders. It is one of the challenging tasks among researchers to determine the proper evaluation of sleep abnormalities during sleep times. Therefore, many approaches were proposed and applied to the sleep stage classification problem. Sleep is an essential requirement for human function, distinguished by alternating behaviors in different body parts such as the brain, muscle, eye, heart, and respiratory activity. It is one of the prerequisites for maintaining both physical and mental health. It incorporates approximately one-third of human life and has a direct relationship with protecting the metabolizable energy, proper functioning of the neuronal system, developing the neuron connections, and building up good memory and learning. As per research findings currently, the lifestyle of people is changing quickly. These changes in lifestyles threaten the disorder of sleeping time, and it ultimately creates different sleep-related diseases in the later period, which significantly affects public safety [1]. Additionally, it has been found from additional demographic reports that up to 24% of the adult population suffered from poor quality sleep for various reasons such as shift duty and a stressful professional life [2]. Apart from that, sometimes unhealthy situations are also responsible for improper sleep during the night, mostly in childhood subjects. In an in-depth study, Ohayon and Smirne found that around 27.6% of the Italian population is affected by sleep-related disorders [3]. According to the Sleep Heart Health Study, it has been found that difficulty in initiating and maintaining sleep and excessive daytime sleepiness have reduced Health-Related Quality of Life (HRQoL) [4]. Some neurological and psychological disorders can sometimes worsen the usual sleep patterns [5]. Some research result analyses signify a cost of more than $100 billion per year [6]. Several researchers found that the average direct and indirect costs of treating sleep-related disorders for six months were approximately $1000. This cost is generally higher than in comparison of normal subjects without sleep problems [7]. Other research has observed a direct link between fatigue and occupational safety [8]. From some clinical assessment, it has been observed that the continuity of sleep problems are statistically linked to poor medical status and worse in socio-professional life [9]. As per the international classification of sleep disorders (ICDS-III) criteria, 83 types of sleep disorders in 7 different sections were defined [10]. Nowadays, some common sleep diseases that affect humans include sleep apnea [11], insomnia [12], bruxism [13], rapid eye movement disorder (RBD) [14], and narcolepsy [15]. This may impact not only our health but also its effects on cognitive functions such as receiving, choosing, transforming, storing, processing, and retrieval of information in the long-term part. To procure the best sleep disorder diagnosis, we first need to analyse the subjects' sleep quality. The crucial part of the diagnosis is to obtain accurate sleep stages monitoring, scoring, and identifying the sleep pattern abnormalities during sleep [16]. The whole night sleep recordings from subjects were processed based on Rechtschaffen & Kales and the American Academy of Sleep Medicine (AASM). According to R&K sleep rules, there are three main sleep stages: wake, non-rapid eye movement (NREM), and rapid eye movement (REM). Further, the NREM sleep stage is divided into four sub-sleep stages: N1, N2, N3, and N4. But according to the AASM standards, the NREM sleep stage is divided into three sub-sleep stages: N1, N2, and N3.

Moreover, the sleep stages proceed cyclically from the NREM to the REM stage, and the cyclic process starts with N1→N2→N3→N2→REM, and the cycle is repeated 4 to 6 times during the whole night of sleep. Each sleep stage characterizes the new A recording to the amplitude, frequency, and shape of the polysomnography (PSG) signals, and the same summary information is shown in Table 1. However, the manual sleep staging scoring is most acceptable in some cases, but it may lead to several pitfalls. One reason is the experience factor of experts, and it is a time-consuming process till the completion of visual inspection labelling; this may lead to some human errors due to long hours of recordings, so it is not convincing for clinicians to obtain a Sleep EEG study [17]. Therefore, automatic sleep scoring is the most effective approach [18]. Many research groups have recently contributed their research work on automating sleep stage classification (sleep scoring analysis). Different signal processing methods and machine learning techniques are obtained to retrieve valuable information from biological signals, such as electroencephalogram (EEG), electrooculogram (EOG), and electromyogram (EMG). Many researchers have used EEG signals to evaluate sleep scores from different sleep stages because EEG is one of the most vital bio-medical signals extracted from the central part of the brain and is ultimately helpful for designing high practical applications in the neurological domain [19]. EEG is a non-invasive procedure, and it extracts the electrical activity of the cerebral cortex of subjects. EEG is evaluated through multiple electrodes which are fixed on the scalp of the patient, and this electrode placement follows 10-20 electrode placement standards and nowadays also followed 10-10 electrode placement which alternatively helps to extract multi-channel EEG signals [12-15]. The EEG signals are segmented into different fixed lengths of segments which are called epochs. Those epochs are to be labelled by sleep experts with standards provided by the American Academy of Sleep Medicine (AASM) or the Rechtschaffen and kales standard [20]. In this proposed study, we have followed AASM for labelling the epoch stages. Each recording time of the EEG signal lasts an average of 8 hours. Therefore, manual interpretation of sleep scoring is quite inconsistent. Hence, the manual approach is limited, and it and calls for an automatic sleep stage classification approach that can automatically measure the sleep score with very high accuracy.

2. Related Work on Sleep Stage Classification

Particular research works were carried out earlier with automated sleep stage scoring algorithms. Generally, most of the contributed works have been designed in different manners. Some researchers have focused upon other domains of feature extraction, and trim work has been proposed with various feature selection techniques. Specific authors have also emphasized adopting different machine learning classification algorithms. Katerina D T. et al. took the ISRUC-sleep dataset for a sleep study, considered a dual channel of EEG signal, and obtained energy features from the input channel. Selected parts are forwarded to the random forest classification system used for sleep stage classification. This model achieved an overall accuracy of 75.29% [21]. Hayat et al. studied a sleep stage classification system based on EEG signals. In this work, the author has used a cyclic alternating pattern (CAP) sleep dataset from the Physio Net repository for these experimental studies. They suggested power spectral density features from the input channel through welch techniques, which help identify the depth range of wave patterns in different frequencies fields. For classification purposes here, the author has used decision tree techniques. An accuracy rate of 81.25% is obtained [22]. Sousa et al. focused extraction of entropy features from respective EEG channels, and temporal features were also extracted to discriminate the properties of input channels. The extracted features are classified with SVM, and it has 86.75% overall accuracy and is subject to sleep stage classification [23]. Hassan, A. R., & Subasi, A. (2017) proposed a methodology for automated sleep staging based on a single channel of EEG signals.

In this work, the EEG signal is first segmented into different frequency sub-bands using tunable-Q wavelet transform (TQWT). The proposed system obtained bootstrap aggregating for classification. The classification model achieved an accuracy of 92.43% for two-state sleep stage classification based on the Sleep-EDF database [24]. Ahnaf Rashik Hassan et al. proposed a system of the empirical model of decomposition techniques for segmenting the EEG signal into different frequency sub-bands. The author has introduced a new classification technique named Random under Sampling boosting (RUSBoost) for classification. The proposed algorithm achieved 98.15% for two-state type [25]. In [26], the authors have used the sleep-EDF datasets for their experimental work, extracted wavelet-based features, and used the neighbourhood component analysis to select the relevant features for the classification process. Here two conventional classifiers were used, such as ANN and SVM, and the author has achieved an overall accuracy of 90.03% and 89.93%, respectively, in a subject to sleep stage classification. In [27], the author has considered a dual channel of EEG signal for sleep scoring evaluation. They have extracted both time-domain and frequency-domain features for distinguishing the abnormality that occurred in different sleep phases. Here they have adopted the Bayesian classifier for the classification purpose of sleep stages and have achieved 83% accuracy in identifying various irregularities during the sleep cycle process.

Generally, sleep is a cyclic approach. Particularly a person can cross through five primary stages while sleeping, including wake (W), non-rapid eye movements (stage N1, stage N2, stage N3), and rapid eye movement (REM) stage. Commonly a sleep cycle goes through different sleep stages. This cyclic process has to be repeated four to five times the whole night, with a period of each cycle taking around 90-120 minutes [28]. Hence, we accept that the sleep stage classification is sequential. Henceforth, we need to consider these sequential characteristics of behavior that occurred during sleep, and this observation can help clinicians monitor the sleep scoring process.

The proposed SleepEEG study is wholly based upon a dual channel of EEG signal and used some conventional machine learning algorithms to discriminate the extracted features between sleep states. Three different classifiers, such as binary support vector machine (SVM), decision tree (DT), and K-nearest neighbor (KNN) algorithm, for classifying the sleep stages.

The critical objective considered in our experimental design:

- Here, we primarily work upon two-state classifications considering multiple EEG signal channels. The primary motivation behind this consideration is to analyze which channel is most effective for sleep scoring analysis.
- The proposed study obtained a machine learning approach to classify extracted time and frequency domain features from respective channels.
- In addition, here, we also compared different adopted machine learning classification algorithms and found which classifier is most potent in the count to analyze sleep stage scoring.

The total contribution of this research work has been segmented into four folds as follows. Section 3 describes the experimental data used in this proposed work. Section 4 describes the methodology obtained for this practical work. Section 5 includes a brief presentation on experimental results and compares the development of the proposed study with earlier contributed work. Finally, Section 6 concludes the proposed research and discusses future work.

3. Experimental Data

To implement the SleepEEG test model, we used the ISRUC-Sleep publicly available dataset to evaluate the proposed objectives. It is a polysomnographic dataset, and it is prepared for sleep researchers. It is an open-access comprehensive dataset for sleep stage classification. This dataset contains the different characteristics oriented subject information, which is more helpful for researchers for their experimental work. ISRUC-Sleep dataset obtained data from adults. Some data has been collected from healthy subjects and few from subjects affected with sleep disorders and issues under a medical condition with the sleep disorder. All those recordings were acquired by the Sleep Medicine Centre of the Hospital of Coimbra University (CHUC) in Portugal during 2009-to 2013 [28]. This dataset categorized the data into three subsections; the first sub-section contains data of 100 adult subjects with information about sleep disorders. Here one session recordings for individual subjects and two sleep experts prepared two hypnograms per particular subject. The second sub-section carried information on only eight issues with symptoms of sleep disorders. In this part, two-session recordings have to be recorded on two different dates for individual subjects. Two hypnogram files must also be maintained as per session recording dates for these recordings.

In the third sub-section, only ten healthy subjects' data are to be contained for one session recording only, and two sleep experts have to prepare two hypnograms for this sub-section category data. This dataset comprised 8-9 hours of whole night polysomnographic (PSGs) recordings from subjects at the sampling rate of 200MHz. In this work, we have used ISRUC-Sleep subsection1 dataset. In this group of data a total of 100 topics are there. Out of that, 53 are male, 42 are female, and five are anonymous. The average age of the subject is 51±16 years, height 1.35±6.63m, weight 65.09±34.97kg, BMI 23.53±12.83kg/m2. All recorded signals from this dataset are generally segmented into 30s epoch lengths. The AASM standard strongly followed all types of operations conducted at recording. This dataset recorded different bio-signals from subjects through 11 electrodes placed in other body parts. This dataset followed 10-20 electrode placement standards for the placement of electrodes in the subject's body.

The collected data from different bio-signals in subsection1 is briefly shown in Table 1. Each epoch was annotated by a sleep specialist with one sleep class stage. Generally, the sleep stages include wake (w), non-rapid eye movement (N1, N2, N3, N4), and rapid eye movement (REM). As per the AASM rule in this study, we have combined N3 and N4 into one stage called N3. The wake and N1 stage is the light sleep state, but the N2 and N3 stage is considered a deep sleep state. Generally, this stage takes 40-60% of total sleep in the cyclic sleep process. In the REM stage, the subject's eye movements happen, and generally, in this phase, dreaming occurs. This sleep state takes around 90-120 minutes in our sleep cycle process. By observing these in balance sleep stages numbers. We also consider two channels to verify which channel data is more effective for sleep scoring. In this study, we have considered two channels, such as C4-A1 and O2-A1, of EEG channels for the experimental work of our SLEEPEEG test model. In this proposed study, we have obtained four subjects from Subgroup-I. ISRUC-Sleep database failures of the ISRUC-Sleep subgroup-I dataset structure are shown in Table 1. The subjects enrolled in this study felt mild sleep problems. Each subject's brain-behavior was monitored and collected through two obtained input channels such as C4-A1 and O2-A. All these recording processes were done as per AASM guidelines and annotated by a sleep expert at a sleep laboratory on a 30s basis. Therefore, each epoch's length is 30s or 3000 samples. The extracted epochs are annotated as wake, N1, N2, N3, and REM. The EEG signal segments description is described in Table 3. Table 4 represents the number of wakes, N1, N2, N3, and REM epochs for all enrolled subjects in this proposed research work database. Each input channel is processed in 30s timeframes in our proposed experiment work. Figure 1, Figure 3, Figure 5, and Figure 7 shows samples of five different stages of sleep with input channel of C4-A1. Similarly, for the O2-A1 channel, the behavior of different stages of sleep patterns are represented in Figure 2, Figure 4, Figure 6, and Figure 8.

Table 1. ISRUC-Sleep Subsection1 Dataset Framework

Polysomnographic Signals	Data Acquisition from different Electrodes Positions
EEG	$EEG_{C3\text{-}A2}$,$EEG_{C4\text{-}A1}$,$EEG_{F3\text{-}A2}$, $EEG_{F4\text{-}A1}$,$EEG_{O1\text{-}A2}$,$EEG_{O2\text{-}A1}$
EOG	$EOG_{LOC\text{-}A2}$,$EOG_{ROC\text{-}A1}$
EMG	EMG_{LEG1},EMG_{LEG2},EMG_{CHIN}

Table 2. Description of epochs of various sleep stages from four subjects used in this study

Sl. No.	Subject Number	Age	Sex	Diagnosis/Other problems
1	Subject-16	50	Male	Sleep Apnea No
2	Subject-18	38	Male	Sleep Apnea PLMS
3	Subject-23	50	Female	Sleep Apnea PLMS
4	Subject-77	46	Female	Sleep Apnea No

4. The Methodology

This research proposes an efficient two-state sleep stage classification based on dual channels. This Sleep EEG test model consists of several steps, and its total workflow is shown in Figure 9. As shown in Figure 9, our proposed research work starts with the signal acquisition from enrolled subjects through dual channels of EEG signal. Once the signal acquisition is over, the pre-processing step is to be obtained to exclude the irrelevant noises and artifacts from recorded tracks, followed by the feature extraction step. Next to the feature selection step is to identify the suitable features for the classification model. Finally, the selected parts are forwarded to different machine learning classification models to evaluate profound abnormality during sleep.

Table 3. Description of epochs of various sleep stages from four subjects used in this study

Subject Number	Wake	N1	N2	N3	REM
16	128 (17.07%)	125 (16.67%)	280 (37.33%)	120 (16.00%)	97 (12.93%)
18	133 (17.73%)	92 (12.27%)	301 (40.13%)	141 (18.80%)	83 (11.07%)
23	212 (28.27%)	99 (13.20%)	270 (36.0%)	65 (8.67%)	104 (13.87%)
77	81 (10.80%)	146 (19.47%)	309 (41.20%)	160 (21.33%)	54 (7.20%)

Table 4. Number of 30s epochs for each sleep stage from one dataset

Dataset Name	Wake	N1	N2	N3	REM	Total
ISRUC SLEEP	554	462	1160	486	338	3000

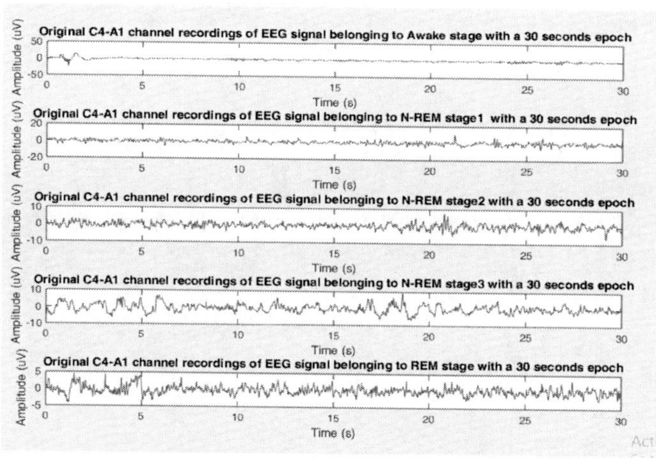

Figure 1. C4-A1 signal in different sleep stages of Subject-16.

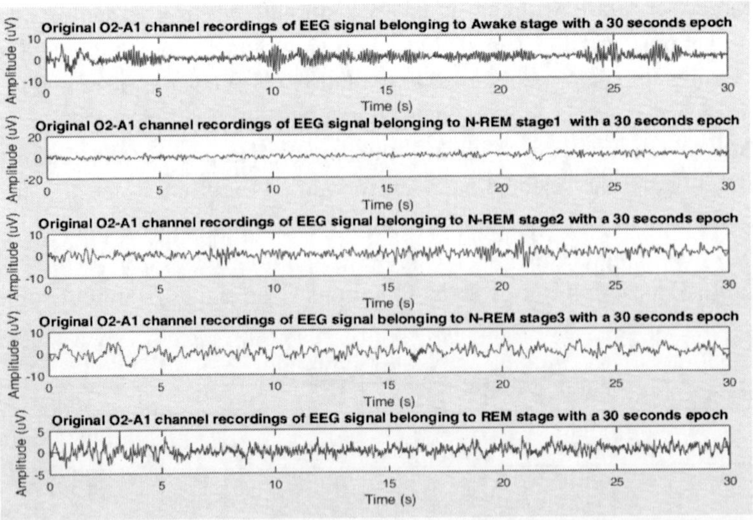

Figure 2. O2-A1 signal in different sleep stages of Subject-16.

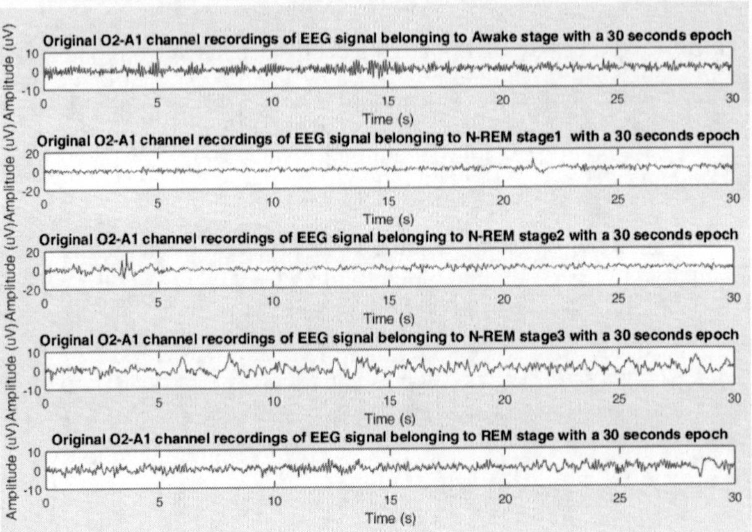

Figure 3. C4-A1 signal in different sleep stages of Subject-18.

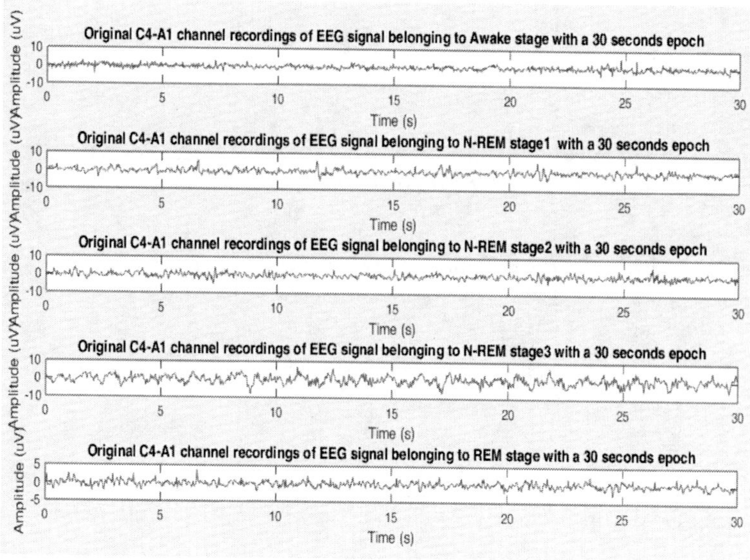

Figure 4. O2-A1 signal in different sleep stages of Subject-18.

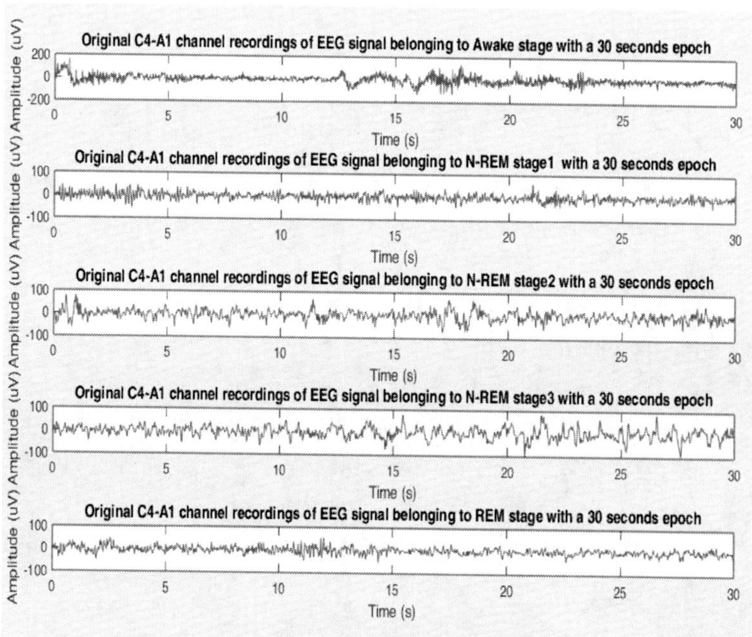

Figure 5. C4-A1 signal in different sleep stages of Subject-23.

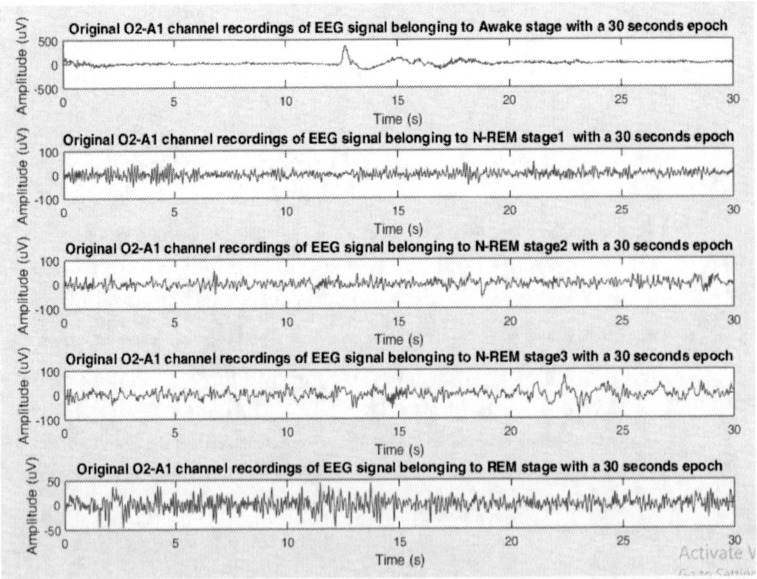

Figure 6. O2-A1 signal in different sleep stages of Subject-23.

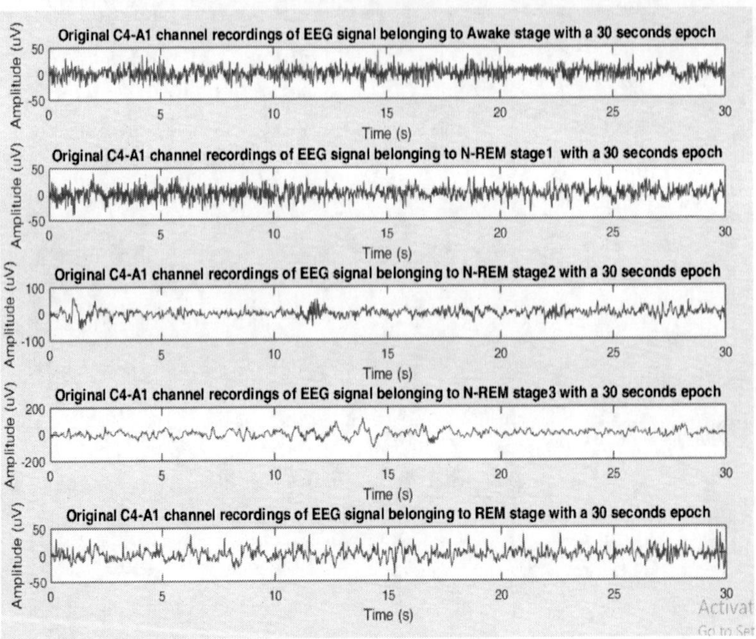

Figure 7. C4-A1 signal in different sleep stages of Subject-77.

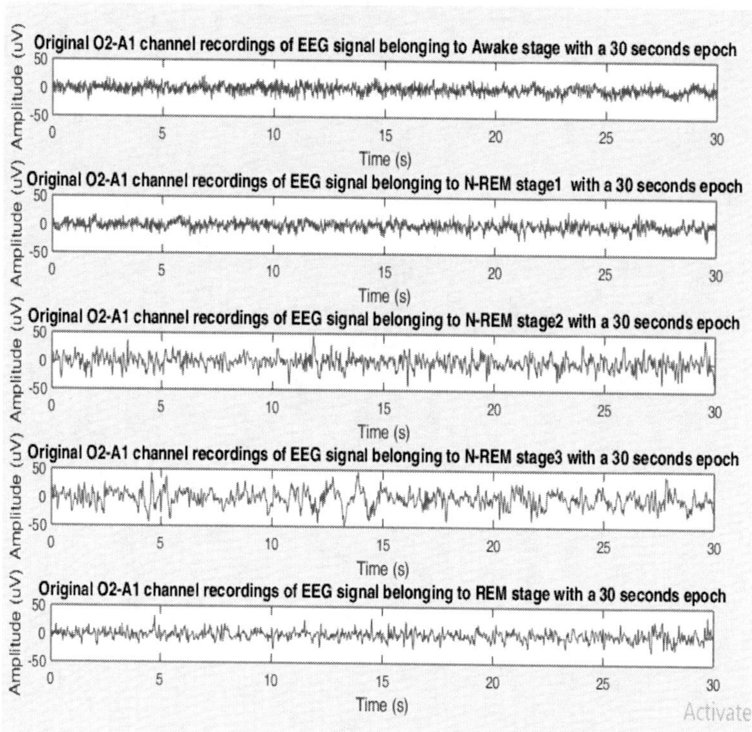

Figure 8. O2-A1 signal in different sleep stages of Subject-77.

4.1. Pre-Processing

In this segment, we briefly present the design and working procedure of our proposed SleepEEG test model. In this work, we have followed the American Academic Standard Medicine (AASM) manuals for all types of operations performed during the sleep stage scoring process.

In this study, we considered a sequence of 30s epochs from the dual channels of EEG signal as input to the SleepEEG test model. First of all, the extracted continuous raw signal has to be segmented into 30s epochs, and each epoch annotated with a proper sleep stage label by referring to the annotation file. Next, we apply the pre-processing techniques to remove the irrelevant noise and artifacts from the primary input signal, which improves the accuracy of identifying the correct score of different sleep stages. In this model, we used Z score normalization. In equation (1), we have mentioned the Z score normalization technique.

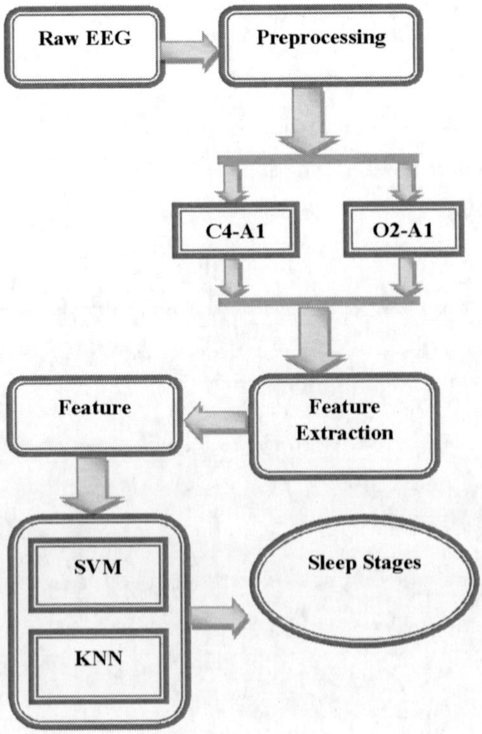

Figure 9. The framework of the proposed research work.

$$V' = (V - \overline{A})/\sigma A \qquad (1)$$

V′, V is new and old for each data entry, respectively. σA is the standard deviation and mean of A, respectively. Next to Z score normalization, we used the 2nd order butter worth filtering techniques to remove the muscle artifacts from the raw signal. The recorded sleep patterns of each enrolled subject before pre-processing and after pre-processing are shown in Table 5, Table 6, Table 7, and Table 8 for subject-16, subject-18, subject-23, and subject-77, respectively.

4.2. Feature Extraction

It is one of the essential parts of the classification model because if the features are not chosen in a healthy manner, it's challenging to identify the irregularities correctly. Ultimately, the classification performance will be degraded. It is also essential to find an effective method for extracting the features from respective obtained input channels. In this proposed study, the recorded signals are segmented into smaller sub-segments, and the size of each segment is the 30s (3000 data points) according to the AASM standards.

Table 5. Analysis of original and filtered channels C4-A1and O2-A1 of EEG signal in subject-16 patient

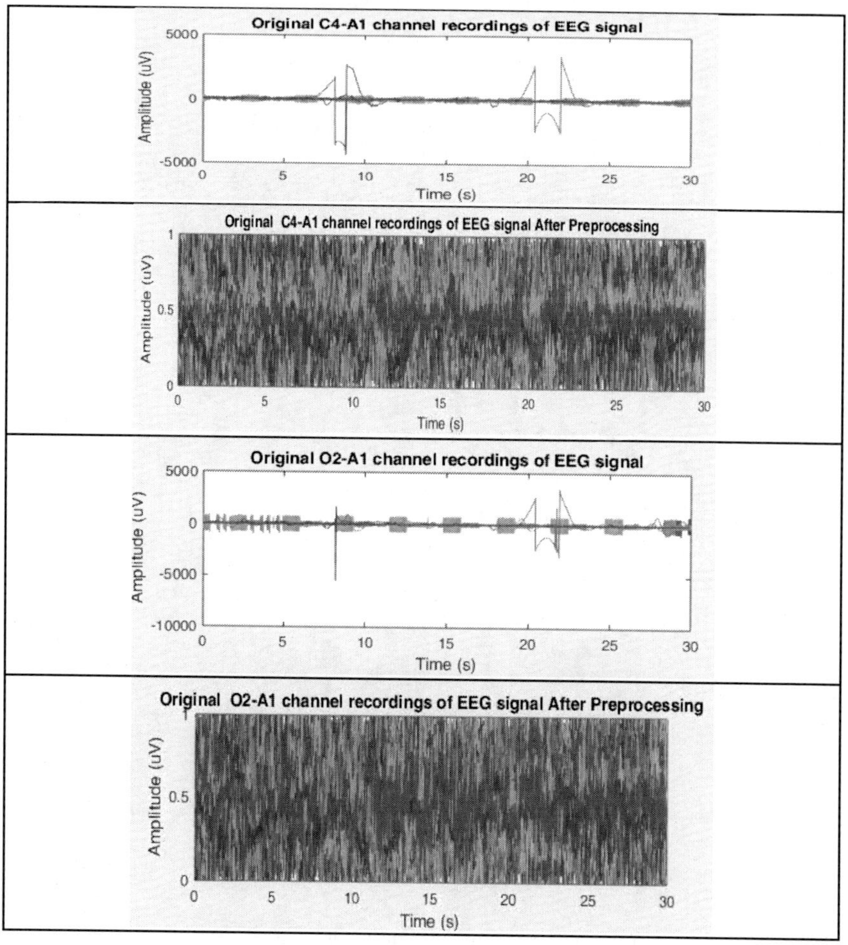

This work extracted 34 features, including time and frequency domain features: 1. six time-domain features 2. twenty-eight frequency domain

features. Henceforth removed features for this research work are briefly described in Table 9.

Table 6. Analysis of original and filtered channel C4-A1 and O2-A1 of EEG signal in subject-18 patient

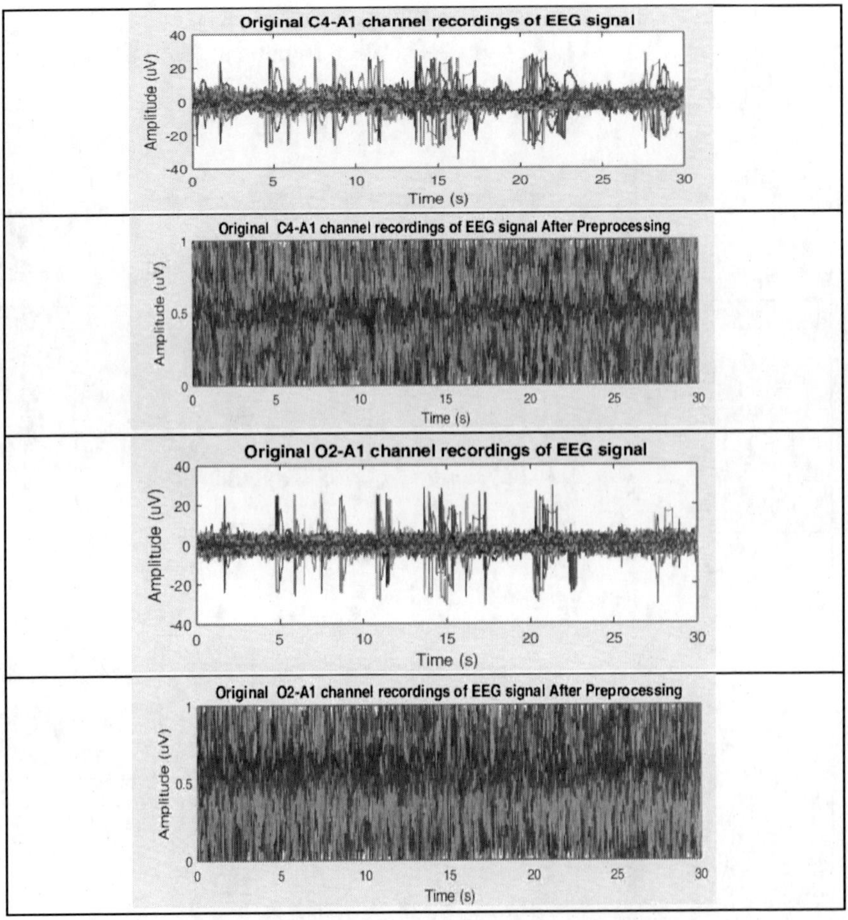

4.3. Feature Selection

Next to feature extraction, we have selected some of the practical features from extracted features which are alternatively helpful for distinguishing the disordered behavior. We have obtained the feature selection techniques to extract the most convenient features. The main aim of this is to get a minimum number of features that are more relevant for discriminating the sleep patterns with adequate accuracy. Also, the feature selection step reduces the over-fitting and computational time to select the appropriate features for classification. Though the PSG-related datasets are large, and we have extracted different types of parts from them, this feature selection step balanced rejecting those features, which has less impact on the evaluation of sleep stage scoring.

Table 7. Analysis of original and filtered channel C4-A1 and O2-A1 of EEG signal in subject-23 patient

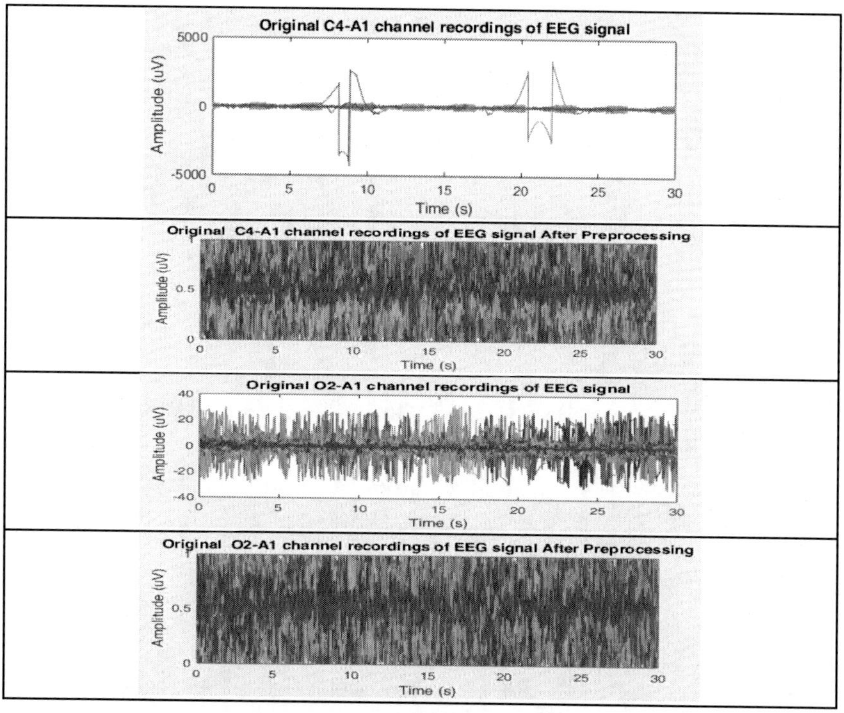

In this study, we have considered the Online Streaming Feature Selection (OSFS) techniques for selecting suitable features for the classification tasks. OSFS divides elements into different categories such as i. powerfully relevant ii. weakly relevant iii. irrelevant features. With this approach, the complete segments are analyzed to find the optimal features set for classification with the help of two phases i) online relevance analysis ii) online redundancy analysis. OSFS discriminates between strong and weak elements in the relevance analysis phase and adds to the Best Candidate Feature (BCF) set. When any new part arrives, OSFS has to verify whether the feature is relevant as per class label value or not, if it satisfies it included with BCF set or discarded. When any new part is added to the BCF set, the relevance phase is performed, ultimately removing the redundant features from the BCF [29].

Table 8. Analysis of original and filtered channel C4-A1 and O2-A1 of EEG signal in subject-77 patient

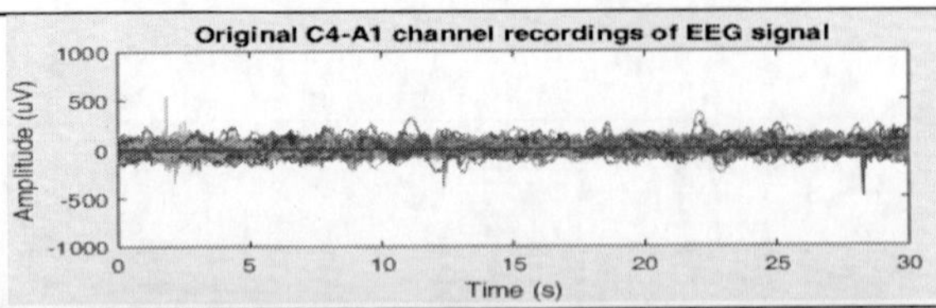

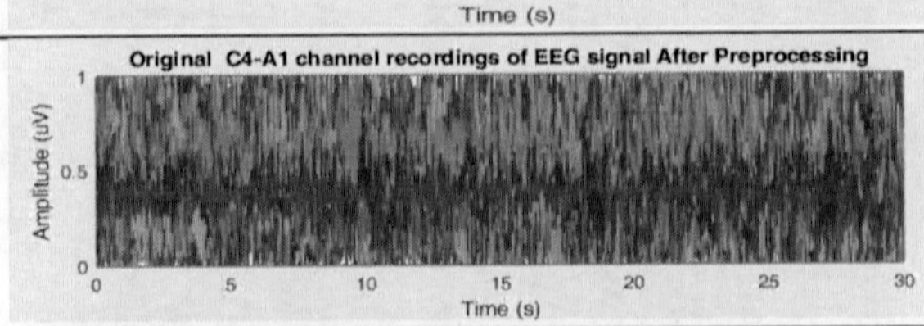

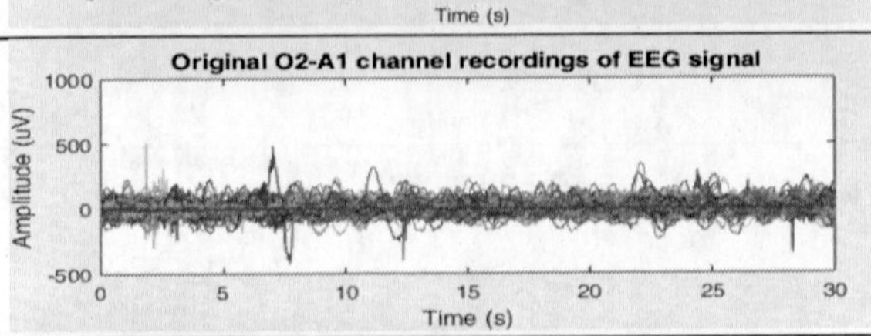

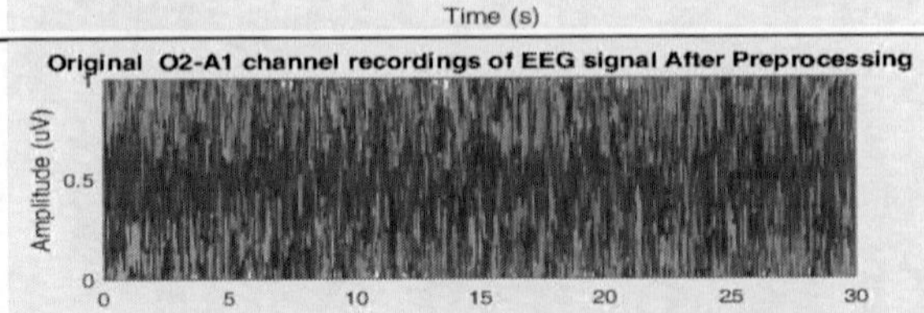

Finally, we have extracted thirty-four features for this experimental study on two-state classifications. In this proposed research work, we have adopted min-max normalization techniques to avoid the effect of EEG features and any abnormal values in the classification process. We made bring all features deals between 0 to 1 only [30]. In equation (2), we have mentioned min-max normalization techniques.

Table 9. Extracted Features for SleepEEG study

Label	Short Narration
F1,F3,F5,F7,F9,F2,F4, F6,F8,F10	Relative Spectral Power(RSP) with different frequency sub-bands
F11,F12,F13	Slow Wave Index for different frequency sub-bands
F14, F15,F16,F17,F18	Centre Frequency(Fc) for different frequency sub-bands
F19,F20,F21,F22,F23	Bandwidth (fσ)
F24,F25,F26,F27,F28	Spectral value at the center frequency (SFC)
F29,F30,F31	Hjorth Parameters
F32	Entropy
F33	Skewness
F34	Kurtosis

Table 10. Selected Features for SleepEEG study

Participants Name/Gender	Channel	Best Feature combination	Classifier
Subject-16 MALE	C4-A1	F1,F2,F3,F4,F5,F7,F9,F10,F11,F13,F14,F15,F22, F25,F27,F31 (16 Features)	SVM KNN
	O1-A2	F1,F2,F3,F4,F5,F7,F11,F12,F15,F16,F17,F20,F24, F26,F31,F33,F37 (17 Features)	SVM KNN
Subject-18 MALE	C4-A1	F1,F2,F3,F4,F5,F7,F8,F9,F11,F12F13,F14,F1,F22,F25 (15 Features)	SVM KNN
	O1-A2	F1,F2,F3,F4,F5,F7,F8,F9,F11,F12F13,F14,F1,F22,F25 (15 Features)	SVM KNN
Subject-23 FEMALE	C4-A1	F1,F2,F3,F4,F5,F7,F8,F9,F10,F11,F15,F16,F18,F27,F2 9,F37 (16 Features)	SVM KNN
	O1-A2	F1,F2,F3,F4,F5,F7,F8,F9,F11,F12F13,F14,F1,F22,F25 (15 Features)	SVM KNN
Subject-77 FEMALE	C4-A1	F1,F2,F3,F4,F5,F7,F8,F9,F11,F12F13,F14,F1,F22,F25 (15 Features)	SVM KNN
	O1-A2	F1,F2,F3,F4,F5,F7,F8,F9,F11,F12F13,F14,F1,F22,F25 (15 Features)	SVM KNN

$$XNorm = [X - \min(X)]/\max(X) - \min(X) \quad (2)$$

Where XNorm represents the feature values after normalization is the initial set of feature values, min and max are the minima and maximum values in the X feature set.

4.4. Classification

After feature selection, we have obtained various classifiers employed to classify selected features and specify a sleep stage for each epoch. This classification model separates the feature vectors into different sleep classes by analysing other classes' linear and non-linear boundaries. This sleeping study has obtained two basic conventional classification techniques for two-state sleep stage classification, such as support vector machine (SVM) and k-nearest neighbor (KNN).

SVM: It is a binary classification technique through which we have analyzed the data and recognized its patterns. SVM considers a set of training samples and designs a model when any new samples test through this trained model; then, the classifier assigns to one class as per its matched characteristics out of the two classes. This condition is only applicable if the problem is a linear separable condition [31].

KNN is one of the base classifiers; this technique is generally obtained in multi-modal distribution-oriented problems only. Our proposed work is exact where the same class of epochs is distributed in different locations in feature vector space. With the help of KNN techniques, we are assigning the labels to those input epochs based on the majority vote of its k-nearest samples [32].

4.5. System Performance Evaluation

In this proposed SleepEEG study, we have adopted some performance metrics to evaluate sleep scoring performances of individual input channels. Besides, we also computed which classification algorithm is more suitable for which channel to be more effective for the sleep scoring process. Additionally, we have considered Cohen's kappa coefficient for measuring the performance of an obtained classifier for classifying the sleep stages. It is more suitable for measuring performances between two classification products. These metrics are defined as follows:

Accuracy = TP +TN/ (TP+TN+FP+FN) [33]
Recall = TP/ (TP+FN) [34]
Specificity = TN/ (TN+FP) [35]
Precision = TP/ (TP+FP) [36]
F1-Score = 2*Precision*Recall / (Precision + Recall) [37]
Kappa Coefficient=2*(TN*TP-FP*FN)

/((TN+FN)*(FN+TP) + (FP+TP) + (TN+FP)) [38]

The two-state sleep stage classification confusion matrix is shown in Table 10. Each row of the confusion matrix represents the instances of an actual class, and each column of the matrix represents instances of the predicted class. Each element location Cij of the confusion matrix is represented between actual class i and predicted class j. The performance evaluation through kappa coefficient has six levels of agreement: 1) poor indication (< 0), 2) slight indication (> 0 to <0.3), 3) fair (0.31 to 0.5), 4) moderate indication (0.51 to 0.7), 5) substantial indication (0.71 to 0.9), and excellent (>0.9) [34].

In this experiment, we have obtained cross-validation techniques to identify the disorder patterns. It is one of the popular techniques subject to pattern validation recognition from feature vectors.

Table 11. Confusion matrix

	Predicted Class	Wake	Sleep
Actual Class	Wake	C_{11}	C_{12}
	Sleep	C_{21}	C_{22}

In this work, we have adopted a k-fold cross-validation technique, and here we employed the k value as ten. It becomes helpful to evaluate the performances of considered classifiers. Here we have used 10-fold cross-validation in which a dataset divided into ten folds equally from that one-fold is taken as a test set and the remaining set to be considered as the training set. At last, all results of the test were combined, and we calculated the classification accuracy. All the experiments have been conducted using an Intel i7-6700 processor with 24 GB RAM for this proposed study. The software is MATLAB R2017a on Windows 10 OS.

5. Experimental Results and Discussion

The main contribution of the proposed study is exploiting channel effectiveness for sleep stage scoring in two-state sleep stage classification. For this implementation work, we have considered two channels. We have enrolled four subjects with different genders, two of them belonging to the male category and the other two belonging to a female type. In this work, we have used dual channels of EEG signals such as C4-A1 and O2-A1 to record the information from considered subjects in this research work. This complete SleepEEG study worked upon the ISRUC-Sleep dataset, which is publicly available online and collected from the Department of Sleep Medicine, Hospital of Coimbra University (CHUC) in Portugal. The entire work of this proposed study follows AASM standard rules to recognize the different sleep patterns. This study has extracted thirty-four features, including both time and frequency domains. In this experimental work, we have used two base classifiers like SVM and KNN, to discriminate between the sleep states.

The primary outcome expected from this contribution are:

1. To find an effective classification algorithm with subjects to best discriminate the abnormality of sleep patterns during sleep hours.
2. To compare channel acquisition effectiveness towards how best to evaluate the sleep scoring.
3. To compare the accuracy between different classifiers to different evaluation metrics to finalize which classification algorithm is more appropriate for detecting the different sleep stages.

Table 12 shows the confusion matrix results of the subject-16 for both the classifiers SVM and KNN. Similarly, Table 13, Table 14, and Table 15 present the confusion matrices achieved by the proposed SleepEEG test model using dual-channel such as C4-A1 and O2-A1 of subject 18, subject 23, and subject 77, respectively.

The performances of each stage of sleep evaluation metrics achieved from each enrolled subject for the C4-A1 channel with SVM and KNN classifier of this SleepEEG study were described briefly in Tables 16 and 17; similarly, for the O2-A1 channel, the evaluation matrices performances with SVM and KNN classifiers are shown in Table 18 and 19 in terms of accuracy, recall, precision, specificity, F1-Score and kappa coefficient. The performance graphs of the proposed SleepEEG test model with the C4-A1 channel of EEG signal for the SVM and KNN classifier are shown in Figure 10 and Figure 11, respectively. Similarly, for the O2-A1 channel, the performances graph representation is shown in Figures 12 and 13. The achieved overall accuracy performances using the C4-A1, and O2-A1 media of EEG signal are shown in Figure 14 and Figure 15. It has been observed from Figure 13, and Figure 14 that the best classification accuracy achieved through the SVM classification model is concerned with the analysis of sleep irregularities during sleep concerning both input channels (C4-A1 and O2-A1). Using an SVM classifier, the proposed Sleep EEG study based on dual channels of EEG signals shows a higher accuracy of 98.53% for subject-77 by C4-A1 input channel; similarly, by using KNN classification techniques, highest accuracy was achieved at 97.07% for subject-77.

Table 12. Confusion matrix performance achieved by the SleepEEG study using C4-A1 and O2-A1 EEG channels from Subject-16

C4-A1		Wake	Sleep
SVM	Wake	302	7
	Sleep	14	427
		Wake	Sleep
KNN	Wake	261	48
	Sleep	48	393
O2-A1		Wake	Sleep
SVM	Wake	185	22
	Sleep	15	528
		Wake	Sleep
KNN	Wake	152	55
	Sleep	44	499

Table 13. Confusion matrix performance achieved by the SleepEEG study using C4-A1 and O2-A1 EEG channels from Subject-18

C4-A1		Wake	Sleep
SVM	Wake	152	18
	Sleep	8	572
		Wake	Sleep
KNN	Wake	126	44
	Sleep	34	556
O2-A1		Wake	Sleep
SVM	Wake	190	24
	Sleep	8	528
		Wake	Sleep
KNN	Wake	169	45
	Sleep	26	510

Specifically, the obtained sensitivity, specificity and F1-score of the C4-A1 channel with SVM classification model from subject 16 is 96.83%, 97.73% and 96.60%, similarly for subject-18, it is 98.62%, 89.41% and 97.78%, for subject-23, it is reached to 96.49%, 94.47% and 95.45% and finally for subject-77, the reported performance is 97.09%, 95.71% and 97.09%.

Table 14. Confusion matrix performance achieved by the SleepEEG study using C4-A1 and O2-A1 EEG channels from Subject-23

C4-A1		Wake	Sleep
SVM	Wake	359	21
	Sleep	13	357
		Wake	Sleep
KNN	Wake	322	58
	Sleep	51	319
O2-A1		Wake	Sleep
SVM	Wake	313	26
	Sleep	10	401
		Wake	Sleep
KNN	Wake	266	73
	Sleep	52	359

Table 15. Confusion matrix performance achieved by the SleepEEG study using C4-A1 and O2-A1 EEG channels from Subject-77

C4-A1		Wake	Sleep
SVM	Wake	290	13
	Sleep	13	434
		Wake	Sleep
KNN	Wake	255	48
	Sleep	43	404
O2-A1		Wake	Sleep
SVM	Wake	497	3
	Sleep	8	242
		Wake	Sleep
KNN	Wake	490	10
	Sleep	12	238

Table 16. The Performance of the Evaluation matrices for the C4-A1 channel through the SVM classification model

C4-A1	Subject 16	Subject 18	Subject 23	Subject 77
Accuracy	97.20%	96.53%	95.47%	96.53%
Precision	98.39%	96.95%	94.44%	97.09%
Sensitivity	96.83%	98.62%	96.49%	97.09%
Specificity	97.73%	89.41%	94.47%	95.71%
F1-Score	97.60%	97.78%	95.45%	97.09%

Table 17. The Performance of the Evaluation matrices for the C4-A1 channel through the KNN classification model

C4-A1	Subject 16	Subject 18	Subject 23	Subject 77
Accuracy	87.17%	89.73%	85.46%	87.87%
Precision	89.07%	92.66%	84.61%	89.38%
Sensitivity	89.07%	94.23%	86.21%	90.38%
Specificity	84.47%	74.11%	85.41%	85.57%
F1-Score	89.07%	93.44%	85.40%	89.87%

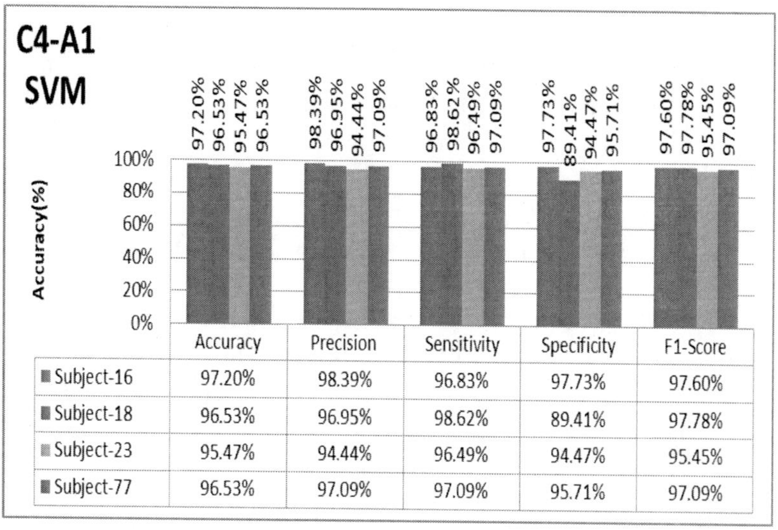

Figure 10. Performance graphs of the proposed SleepEEG test model with the C4-A1 channel of EEG signal for the SVM classifier.

Similarly, for KNN classification model, the specified parameters reached to 89.07%, 84.47% and 89.07% for subject-16, 94.23%, 74.11% and 93.44% for subject-23, 86.21%, 85.4%, 85.40% for subject-23 and at last for subject - 77 it is 90.38%, 85.57% and 89.87%. Meanwhile, the obtained sensitivity, specificity and F1-Score for O2-A1 channel with SVM model was 97.24%, 89.37% and 96.61% for subject-16, 98.51%, 88.79% and 97.06% for subject-18, 97.57%, 92.33% and 95.70% for subject-23, 95.20%, 98.00% and 95.88% for subject-77. Similarly, the performance of obtained sensitivity, specificity and F1-Score for O2-A1 channel with KNN classification system is 91.90%, 73.43% and 90.98% for subject-16, 95.14%, 78.97%, 93.49% for subject-18, 87.35%, 83.68% and 85.17% for subject-23, 95.20%, 98.0% and 95.58% for subject-77. Table 20 and 21 present the average accuracy and kappa coefficient for Subject-16 for the C4-A1 and O2-A1 channels through the SVM and KNN classification models. Similarly, Table 22 and Table 23 for subject-18, Table 24 and Table 25 for subject-23, and finally Table 26 and Table 27 for subject-77. In our proposed research work, the SVM classification techniques turned out to be most useful for classifying the sleep stages of subject-16 through the C4-A1 channel with an accuracy of 97.20% and kappa coefficient of 1.88, similarly for the O2-A1 channel with an accuracy of 98.53% and kappa coefficient of 1.92, which indicates a substantial agreement with the gold standard. Another significance of our proposed research work is that, to the best of our knowledge, this is the unique method for sleep stage classification based on dual channels of EEG signal. SleepEEG study provides a new aspect of sleep stage scoring with an analysis of two types of features of sleep stages where one feature represents the signal changes in different sleep stages during sleep. For example, the NREM patterns have mixed frequency behavior, and SWS has a lower frequency. The other feature tracked dynamic behavior during night sleep time. It can help discover new things subject to sleep stage analysis. It may help for best prediction towards sleep irregularities during sleep and ultimately advantages the healthcare sector for diagnosis of sleep-related diseases.

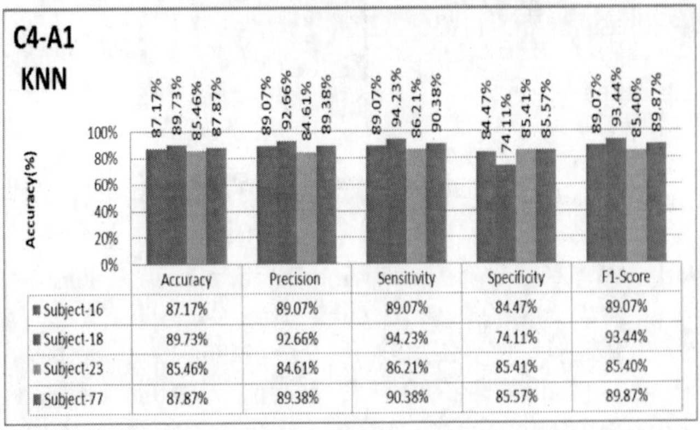

	Accuracy	Precision	Sensitivity	Specificity	F1-Score
Subject-16	87.17%	89.07%	89.07%	84.47%	89.07%
Subject-18	89.73%	92.66%	94.23%	74.11%	93.44%
Subject-23	85.46%	84.61%	86.21%	85.41%	85.40%
Subject-77	87.87%	89.38%	90.38%	85.57%	89.87%

Figure 11. Performance graphs of the proposed SleepEEG test model with the C4-A1 channel of EEG signal for the KNN classifier.

Our proposed study has some limitations: 1) only a dual channel of EEG signal was used to analyze sleep stages 2) we have not considered concepts of some sleep-related disorders such as bruxism, narcolepsy, and insomnia, on their influences on classification. In future work, we will concentrate on including more channels of EEG signals and PSG signals such as EMG, EOG, and ECG to improve the accuracy of our proposed SleepEEG study. Additionally, we will focus on designing some optimization algorithm that helps select the appropriate features for the classification model. We will also consider more datasets in our future research work implementations.

To analyze the performance of the proposed research work, we compared our suggested research classification results with those of four other reported methods. The table shows that the version of the proposed research work is more accurate than other contribution work.

Table 18. The Performances of the Evaluation matrices for the O2-A1 channel through the SVM classification model

O2-A1	Subject 16	Subject 18	Subject 23	Subject 77
Accuracy	95.07%	95.73%	95.20%	98.53%
Precision	96.00%	95.65%	93.91%	98.78%
Sensitivity	97.24%	98.51%	97.57%	96.80%
Specificity	89.37%	88.79%	92.33%	99.40%
F1-Score	96.61%	97.06%	95.70%	97.78%

Table 19. The Performance of the Evaluation matrices for the O2-A1 channel through the KNN classification model

O2-A1	Subject 16	Subject 18	Subject 23	Subject 77
Accuracy	86.80%	90.53%	83.00%	97.06%
Precision	90.07%	91.89%	83.10%	95.97%
Sensitivity	91.90%	95.14%	87.35%	95.20%
Specificity	73.43%	78.97%	83.65%	98.00%
F1-Score	90.98%	93.49%	85.17%	95.58%

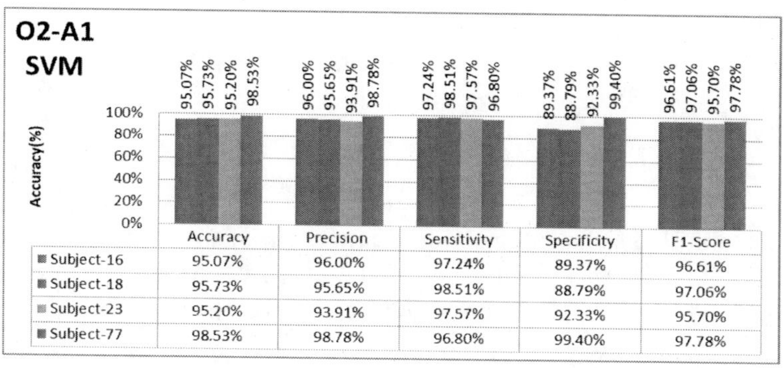

Figure 12. Performance graphs of the proposed SleepEEG test model with the O2-A1 channel of EEG signal for the SVM classifier.

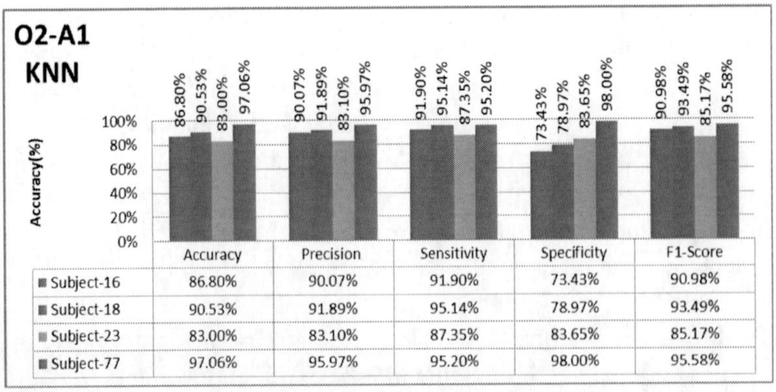

Figure 13. Performance graphs of the proposed SleepEEG test model with the O2-A1 channel of EEG signal for the KNN classifier.

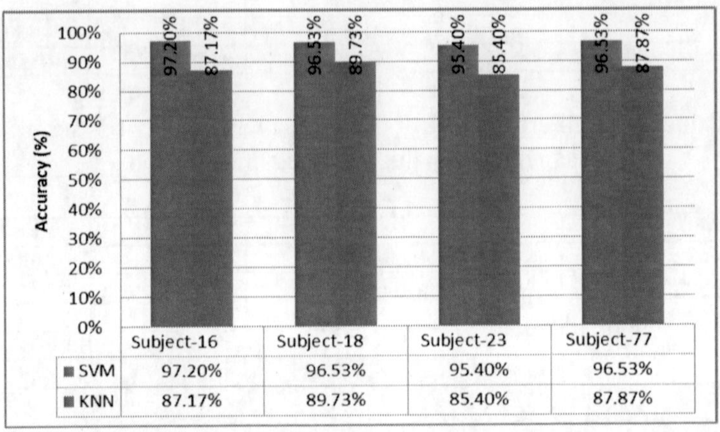

Figure 14. Graphs of performances obtained accuracy C4-A1 channel of EEG signal.

Conclusion

In the present study, we have designed a SleepEEG test model using dual channels of EEG signal. Current research work has only enrolled four subjects of a different gender for our experimental work. We have presented a novel comparison of channel effectiveness in the count to sleep scoring of sleep stages. Additionally, we also compared classification algorithm performance in this study, and we found that the SVM classifier is most suitable for sleep stage scoring with higher accuracy incomparable to the KNN classifier. The proposed features from the time and frequency domain provided valuable information to analyze the changes in the behavior of sleep stages. SVM classifier and C4-A1 channel were more suitable for getting high accuracy sleep stage scoring from EEG signal recordings. Table 28 presents that our proposed SleepEEG study is significantly better than previous contributions by giving a higher accuracy for the sleep stage scoring assignment. While designing the automated sleep stage classification model, there may be data imbalance problems that sometimes occurred in between standard class data versus disease class data. This problem we will solve with our future work through new techniques. Our developed SleepEEG study can be applied to so many biomedical applications and clinical systems to diagnose neurological disorders.

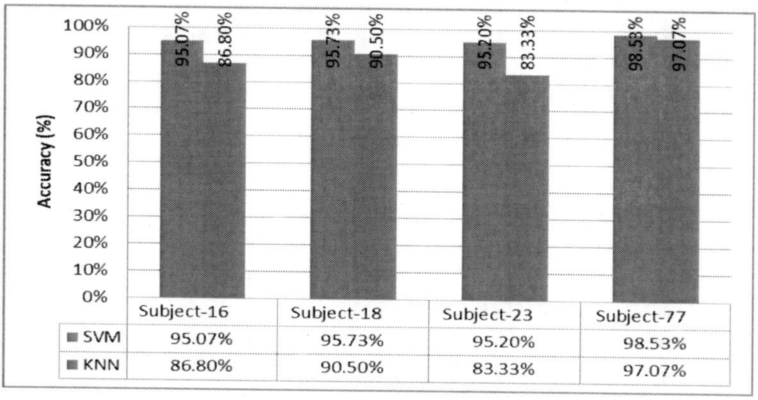

Figure 15. Graphs of performances obtained accuracy O2-A1 channel of EEG signal.

Table 20. The average accuracy and kappa coefficient for Subject-16 for both the C4-A1 and O2-A1 channel through the SVM classification model

Subject-16 SVM Classifier	C4-A1		O2-A1	
Sleep Stages	**Accuracy Rate**	**Kappa coefficient**	**Accuracy Rate**	**Kappa coefficient**
Wake	97.20%	1.91	95.07%	1.69
Sleep	97.20%	1.84	95.07%	1.78
Average	97.20%	1.88	95.07%	1.74

Table 21. The average accuracy and kappa coefficient for Subject-16 for both the C4-A1 and O2-A1 channel through the KNN classification model

Subject-16 KNN Classifier	C4-A1		O2-A1	
Sleep Stages	Accuracy Rate	Kappa coefficient	Accuracy Rate	Kappa coefficient
Wake	87.17%	1.46	86.80%	1.27
Sleep	87.17%	1.46	86.80%	1.37
Average	87.17%	1.46	86.80%	1.32

Table 22. The average accuracy and kappa coefficient for Subject-18 for both the C4-A1 and O2-A1 channel through the SVM classification model

Subject-18 SVM Classifier	C4-A1		O2-A1	
Sleep Stages	Accuracy Rate	Kappa coefficient	Accuracy Rate	Kappa coefficient
Wake	96.53%	1.71	95.73%	1.68
Sleep	96.53%	1.85	86.80%	1.87
Average	96.53%	1.78	91.27%	1.78

Table 23. The average accuracy and kappa coefficient for Subject-18 for both the C4-A1 and O2-A1 channel through the KNN classification model

Subject-18 KNN Classifier	C4-A1		O2-A1	
Sleep Stages	Accuracy Rate	Kappa coefficient	Accuracy Rate	Kappa coefficient
Wake	96.53%	1.71	90.53%	1.42
Sleep	96.53%	1.85	90.53%	1.61
Average	96.53%	1.78	90.53%	1.52

Table 24. The average accuracy and kappa coefficient for Subject-23 for both the C4-A1 and O2-A1 channel through the SVM classification model

Subject-23 SVM Classifier	C4-A1		O2-A1	
Sleep Stages	Accuracy Rate	Kappa coefficient	Accuracy Rate	Kappa coefficient
Wake	95.46%	1.77	95.20%	1.72
Sleep	95.46%	1.84	95.20%	1.87
Average	95.46%	1.81	95.20%	1.80

Table 25. The average accuracy and kappa coefficient for Subject-23 for both the C4-A1 and O2-A1 channel through the KNN classification model

Subject-23 KNN Classifier	C4-A1		O2-A1	
Sleep Stages	Accuracy Rate	Kappa coefficient	Accuracy Rate	Kappa coefficient
Wake	85.46%	1.38	83.33%	1.24
Sleep	85.46%	1.43	83.33%	1.39
Average	85.46%	1.41	83.33%	1.32

Table 26. The average accuracy and kappa coefficient for Subject-77 for both the C4-A1 and O2-A1 channel through the SVM classification model

Subject-77 SVM Classifier	C4-A1		O2-A1	
Sleep Stages	Accuracy Rate	Kappa coefficient	Accuracy Rate	Kappa coefficient
Wake	96.53%	1.84	98.53%	1.95
Sleep	96.53%	1.84	98.53%	1.89
Average	96.53%	1.84	98.53%	1.92

Table 27. The average accuracy and kappa coefficient for Subject-77 for both the C4-A1 and O2-A1 channel through the KNN classification model

Subject-77 KNN Classifier	C4-A1		O2-A1	
Sleep Stages	Accuracy Rate	Kappa coefficient	Accuracy Rate	Kappa coefficient
Wake	87.87%	1.46	97.07%	1.86
Sleep	87.87%	1.50	97.07%	1.84
Average	87.87%	1.48	97.07%	1.85

Table 28. Comparison results of proposed work with the previous contribution work with different obtained sleep datasets

Authors Year	Dataset	Name of the Classifier	Features Used	Accuracy
Sousa et al. [23] 2015	ISRUC Sleep	SVM	Entropy Features Skewness, Kurtosis	86.75%
Katerina et al. [21] 2018	ISRUC Sleep	Random Forest	Energy	75.29%
Alizadeh Savareh et al. [26]	Physionet Sleep-EDF	SVM	Energy	89.93%
2018		ANN		90.30%
Heyat et al. [22] 2019	Physionet Sleep-CAP	Decision Tree	Power Spectral Density	81.25%
Proposed Work	ISRUC Sleep	SVM	Hjorth Parameter Spectral Power, Centre Frequency, Bandwidth, Harmonic Parameters Wave Index, Kurtosis, Entropy, Skewness	97.20%
2020		KNN		96.53%

References

Alizadeh Savareh, B., Bashiri, A., Behmanesh, A., Meftahi, G. H., and Hatef, B. (2018). 'Performance comparison of machine learning techniques in sleeps scoring based on wavelet features and neighboring component analysis'. *PeerJ* 6:e5247.

Bajaj, V., and R. B. Pachori, "Automatic classification of sleep stages based on the time-frequency image of EEG signals," *Comput. Methods Programs Biomed.,* vol. 112, no. 3, pp. 320–328, 2013.

Baldwin, C. M., Griffith, K. A., Nieto, F. J., O'Connor, G. T., Walsleben, J. A., & Redline, S. (2001). The Association of Sleep-Disordered Breathing and Sleep Symptoms with Quality of Life in the Sleep Heart Health Study. *Sleep,* 24(1), 96–105.

Berry R. B., Brooks R., Gamaldo C. E., Hardsim S. M., Lloyd R. M., Marcus C. L., Vaughn B. V. *The AASM manual for the scoring of sleep and associated events: rules, terminology and technical specifications,* version 2.1. Darien: American Academy of Sleep Medicine; 2014.

Berry, R. B. Brooks, R., Gamaldo, C. E. Harding, S. M., Marcus, C., and Vaughn, B., (2012) '*The AASM manual for the scoring of sleep and associated events*', Rules, Terminology and Technical Specifications, Darien, Illinois, American Academy of Sleep Medicine.

Boostani, R., Karimzadeh, F., and Nami, M. (2017) 'A comparative review on sleep stage classification methods in patients and healthy individuals', *Comput. Methods Programs Biomed,* Vol. 140, pp.77–91.

Chiu, C. C., Hai, B. H., & Yeh, S. J. (2014). 'Recognition of sleep stages based on a combined neural network and fuzzy system using wavelet transform features'. *Biomedical Engineering: Applications, Basis and Communications,* Vol. 26, No. 02.

Fabien, Lauer. Yann, Guermeur., Mpack, M. S. V., A Multi-Class Support Vector Machine Package. *Journal of Machine Learning Research.* 12,2293-2296(2011).

Fulgencio, L. Corrêa-Faria, P., Lage, C. Paiva, S., Pordeus, I. and Serra-Negra, J. (2016) 'Diagnosis of sleep bruxism can assist in the detection of cases of verbal school bullying and measure the life satisfaction of adolescents', *International Journal of Pediatric Dentistry,* vol. 27, pp.293-301

Hassan, A. R., & Bhuiyan, M. I. H. (2017). Automated identification of sleep states from EEG signals by means of ensemble empirical mode decomposition and random under sampling boosting. *Computer Methods and Programs in Biomedicine,* 140, 201–210.

Hassan, A. R., & Subasi, A. (2017). A decision support system for automated identification of sleep stages from single-channel EEG signals. *Knowledge-Based Systems,* 128, 115–124.

Heyat, M., B. B., Lai, D., and Zhang, F. I. K. Y. (2019). 'Sleep Bruxism Detection Using Decision Tree Method by the Combination of C4-P4 and C4-A1 Channels of Scalp EEG'. *IEEE Access,* Vol. 1–1.

Hsu, Y. L., Y. T. Yang, J. S. Wang, and C. Y. Hsu, "Automatic sleep stage recurrent neural classifier using energy features of EEG signals," *Neurocomputing,* vol. 104, pp. 105–114, Mar. 2013.

Khalighi, S., Sousa, T., Santos, J. M., & Nunes, U. (2016). ISRUC-Sleep: A comprehensive public dataset for sleep researchers. Computer Methods and Programs in Biomedicine, 124, 180–192.

Léger, D., Guilleminault, C., Bader, G., Lévy, E., & Paillard, M. (2002). Medical and Socio-Professional Impact of Insomnia. *Sleep,* 25(6), 621–625.

Liang, S. F., C. E. Kuo, Y. H. Hu, and Y. S. Cheng, "A rule-based automatic sleep staging method," *Journal of neuroscience methods,* vol. 205, no. 1, pp. 169–176, 2012.

Liu, X., Y, Yan., L., Zeng, B., and Wang, W. (2010) 'Automatic sleep stage scoring using Hilbert–Huang transform with BP neural network', In *Proceedings of the 4th International Conference on Bioinformatics and Biomedical Engineering (iCBBE),* 18–20 June 2010. Chengdu, China.

Malhotra, A., Younes, M., Kuna, S. T., Benca, R., Kushida, C. A., Walsh, J., Hanlon, A., Staley, B., Pack, A. I., and Pien, G. W. (2013) 'Performance of an Automated Polysomnography Scoring System Versus Computer-Assisted Manual Scoring'. *Sleep,* Vol. 4, pp. 573-582.

Masaaki, Hanaoka., Masaki, Kobayashi., Haruaki, Yamazaki., Automated Sleep Stage Scoring by Decision Tree Learning. *Proceedings of the 23rd Annual EMBS International Conference,* October 25-28, Istanbul, Turkey, 2001.

Masaaki, Hanaoka., Masaki, Kobayashi., Haruaki, Yamazaki., Automated Sleep Stage Scoring by Decision Tree Learning. *Proceedings of the 23rd Annual EMBS International Conference,* October 25-28, Istanbul, Turkey, 2001.

Ohayon, M. M. (2002) Epidemiology of insomnia: what we know and what we still need to learn. *Sleep Medicine Reviews,* 6(2), 97–111.

Ohayon, M. M., & Smirne, S. (2002). Prevalence and consequences of insomnia disorders in the general population of Italy.

Ozminkowski, R. J., Wang, S., & Walsh, J. K. (2007). The Direct and Indirect Costs of Untreated Insomnia in Adults in the United States. *Sleep,* 30(3), 263–273.

Piñero, P., Garcia, P., Arco, L., Álvarez, A., García, M. M., & Bonal, R. (2004). 'Sleep stage classification using fuzzy sets and machine learning techniques', *Neurocomputing,* Vol. 58-60, pp.1137–1143.

Rahman, Farook, Heyat, and Siddiqui. (2016) 'An Overview of Narcolepsy', *International Advanced Research Journal in Science, Engineering and Technology,* vol. 3, pp. 85-87.

Sanders, T. H., M. McCurry, and M. A. Clements, "Sleep stage classification with cross frequency coupling," in *Proc. 36th Annu. Int. Conf. IEEE Eng. Med. Biol. (EMBC),* Aug. 2014, pp. 4579–4582.

Sateia., Michael, J. (2014) 'International Classification of Sleep Disorders', *Journal of the American College of Chest Physicians,* Vol.146, pp.1387-1394.

Sharmaa, Manish., Mitesh, Ravala., and Acharya, Rajendra U. (2019) 'A new approach to identify obstructive sleep apnea using an optimal orthogonal wavelet filter bank with ECG signals', *Informatics in Medicine Unlocked,* Vol. 16 [online].

Siddiqui, M., Srivastava, G. and Saeed, S. (2016) 'Diagnosis of insomnia sleep disorder using short time frequency analysis of PSD approach applied on EEG signal using channel ROC-LOC', *Sleep Science,* vol. 9, pp.186-191.

Sim, J., and C. C. Wright, "The kappa statistic in reliability studies: use, interpretation, and sample size requirements," *Physical therapy,* vol. 85, no. 3, pp. 257–268, 2005.

Sousa, T., Cruz, A., Khalighi, S., Pires, G., and Nunes, U. (2015). 'A two-step automatic sleep stage classification method with dubious range detection'. *Computers in Biology and Medicine,* Vol. 59, pp. 42–53.

Tzimourta, K. D., Tsilimbaris, A., Tzioukalia, K., Tzallas, A. T., Tsipouras, M. G., Astrakas, L. G., and Giannakeas, N. (2018) 'EEG-Based Automatic Sleep Stage Classification', *Biomedical Journal of Scientific & Technical Research,* Vol. 7 (4).

Wickwire, E. M., Shaya, F. T., & Scharf, S. M. (2016). Health economics of insomnia treatments: The return on investment for a good night's sleep. *Sleep Medicine Reviews,* 30, 72–82.

Willemen, T., VanDeun, D., Verhaert, V., Vandekerckhove, M., Exadaktylos, V., Verbraecken, J., Vander Sloten, J. (2014) An Evaluation of Cardiorespiratory and Movement Features With Respect to Sleep-Stage Classification. *IEEE Journal of Biomedical and Health Informatics,* 18(2), 661–669.

Williamson, A., Lombardi, D. A., Folkard, S., Stutts, J., Courtney, T. K., & Connor, J. L. (2011). The link between fatigue and safety. *Accident Analysis & Prevention,* 43(2), 498–515.

Younes, M. (2017) 'The case for using digital EEG analysis in clinical sleep medicine'. *Sleep Science Practice* 1:2.

Zibrandtsen I., Kidmose P., Otto M., Ibsen J., Kjaer T. W. Case comparison of sleep features from ear-EEG and scalp-EEG. *Sleep Sci.* 2016; 9(2):69–72.

About the Editors

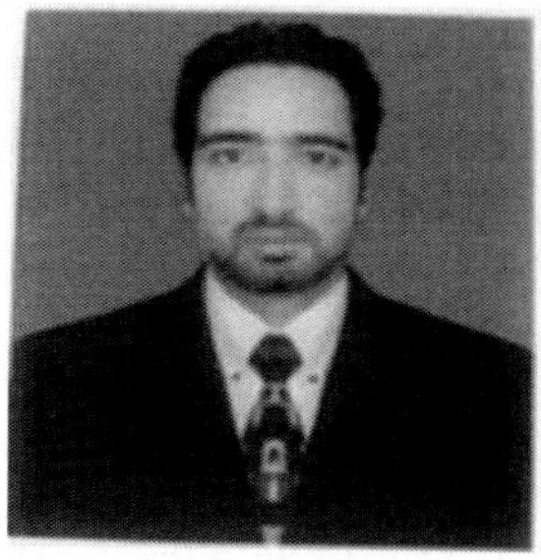

1: Dr. Tawseef Ayoub Shaikh is working as an Assistant Professor in the Department of Computer Science & Engineering, Pandit Deendayal Energy University, India. He obtained his Ph.D. as a full-time Visvesvaraya fellow (MeitY, GoI), from Aligarh Muslim University, Uttar Pradesh, India in 2020. He has published more than 20 papers in journals of National & International repute. He has completed four projects from NPIU MHRD, two as PI, and two as Co-PI with a budget of 16 lakh INR, in collaboration with IIT Indore. He is working as Co-PI in collaboration with NIT Srinagar on two projects granted by JKSTIC worth 9 lakhs INR. He has a total of 4 years of teaching experience and 10 years of research experience. **ORCID: 0000-0003-1433-6181**

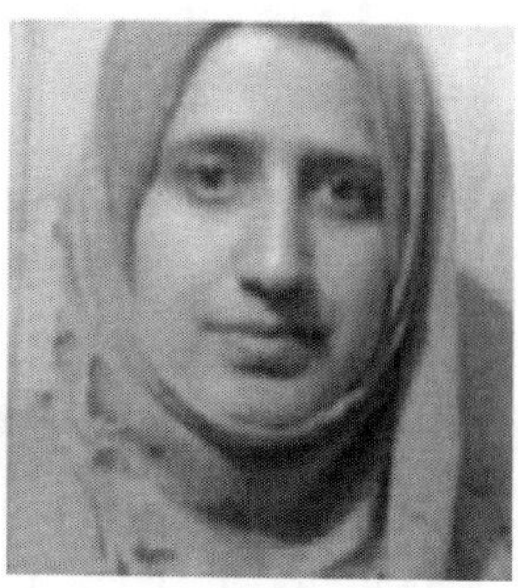

2: Dr. Tabasum Rasool is a Research Associate at the Interdisciplinary Center for Water Research at the Indian Institute of Science, Bangalore. She has completed her Ph.D. in Civil Engineering from the National Institute of Technology, Srinagar. She received her B.tech in Agricultural Engineering from the Sher-e-Kashmir University of Agricultural Sciences and Technology, Kashmir, India in 2012, and M. tech in land and water management from the Sher-e-Kashmir University of Agricultural Sciences and Technology, Kashmir, India in 2014. Currently, her research interests include GIS, climate change, hydrological modeling, vadose zone modeling, groundwater modeling, and integrated water resources management, and she is focused on studying the impact of temperature extremes on rainfall events. She has published more than 12 papers in reputed journals and conferences.

ORCID: 0000-0002-2282-7952

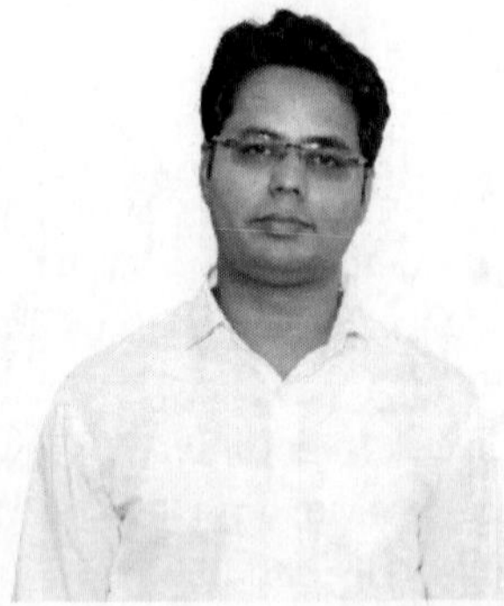

3: Dr. Mohammed Wasid is currently working as an Assistant Professor in the Interdisciplinary Centre for Artificial Intelligence at the Aligarh Muslim University, Aligarh, India. He received his Ph.D. degree in Computer Engineering from Zakir Hussain College of Engineering and Technology, Aligarh Muslim University, Aligarh, India. He has about five years of teaching experience and eight years of research experience. He has published several articles in International Journals, Conferences and Book Chapters which are indexed in reputed indexing bodies like SCI, SCIE, WoS, Scopus. Dr. Mohammed Wasid has qualified national level exams in Computer Science Engineering like UGC-NET and GATE. He has been granted four fully funded research projects by MHRD, NPIU, GoI and he has completed all of them in the capacity of Investigator and Co-investigator. He has been the MANF fellow during his PhD which is the prestigious fellowship granted by UGC, Government of India. His current areas of research are Web Personalization, Machine Learning, and Computational Web Intelligence.

ORCID: 0000-0002-7408-6455

List of Contributors

Akib Mohi Ud Din Khanday
Qamar Rayees Khan
Syed Tanzeel Rabani
Rumaan Bashir
Mahmood Hussain Mir
Sanjay Jamwal
Shahidul Islam
Waseem Ahmad Mir
Izharuddin
Tawseef Ayoub Shaikh
Junaid Ali Reshi
Ayushi Chahal
Preeti Gulia
Nasib Singh Gill
M. Deepika
D. Karthika
Anjume Shakir
E. Fantin Irudaya Raj
Nayana Gupta
N. Manoj Kumar
Deepak Kumar Bagchi
Tabasum Rasool
Abrar Rasool
Santosh Kumar Satapathy
Debabrata Swain
Rupalin Nanda

Index

D

E

F

J

K

L

N

O

P

S

T

U

V

W

X

Y